"An inspiring and informative approach to health.
It combines a profound respect for the innate intelligence
of the human body with a clear exposition of how
to cooperate with its healing power with minimal
yet precise intervention."
—*Timothy Gallwey, author of* The Inner Game of Tennis
and The Inner Game of Work

"As president of the Palmer Chiropractic Colleges
(a system that includes the world's first and largest
chiropractic college and the "Fountainhead of
Chiropractic") I am committed to working with individuals
such as Dr. Lenarz to bring a health care revolution
into being in our lifetimes. It is our responsibility
to speak loudly and clearly to the issue.
This book does so beautifully."
—*Guy F. Riekeman, D.C.*

"Even though I consider myself to be open-minded, it took
my thumb going numb (not a good thing for a surgeon)
for me to consider chiropractic. Chiropractic treatments
resulted in full return of sensation—and have helped to
resolve aches and pains that I thought were just part of
aging. Chiropractic has been a very good thing for me,
and I believe Dr. Lenarz's book is a great way of
introducing it to other people."
—*Kenneth L. Stein, M.D., plastic and reconstructive surgeon*

THE CHIROPRACTIC WAY

How Chiropractic Care Can Stop Your Pain and Help You Regain Your Health Without Drugs or Surgery

Michael Lenarz, D.C.

with

Victoria St. George

B A N T A M   B O O K S
New York Toronto London Sydney Auckland

THE CHIROPRACTIC WAY

A Bantam Book

PUBLISHING HISTORY

Bantam trade paperback edition / April 2003

Published by Bantam Dell

A Division of Random House, Inc.
New York, New York

BOOK DESIGN BY GLEN EDELSTEIN

Library of Congress Cataloging in Publication Data
Lenarz, Michael, D. C.
The chiropractic way: how chiropractic care can stop your
pain and help you regain your health without drugs or
surgery / Michael Lenarz with Victoria St. George.
—Bantam trade pbk. ed.
p. cm.
Includes bibliographical references.
ISBN 0-553-38159-8
1. Chiropractic—Popular works. 2. Pain—Alternative treatment—Popular works.   I. St. George, Victoria.   II. Title.
RZ244.L46 2003
615.5'34—dc21
2002043792

Manufactured in the United States of America

Published simultaneously in Canada

RRH 10 9 8 7 6 5 4 3 2 1

To Prem Rawat,
who has taught me about myself.
—Michael

Over the past fifteen years, I have seen the benefits of chiropractic care in thousands of patients in my practice, and I have drawn on their stories throughout this book. When I have based case histories on particular patients, I have changed their names and distinguishing features to preserve their privacy.

The Chiropractic Way is designed to serve as your guide to a more holistic approach to health maintenance, and to the treatment of health conditions and diseases. However, the suggestions and examples it presents are not prescriptive. No health care practitioner would recommend a course of care unless he or she knew the details of a patient's health. My goal is to give you the information you need to make informed choices.

Do not self-diagnose. If you have symptoms that suggest an illness described in this book, please consult your health care professional. If you are currently taking prescription medications, it is important not to discontinue any drug or alter your drug regimen without consulting your provider.

It is my sincere hope that you—or someone you care about—will use the information provided in the following pages to achieve greater health and happiness.

TABLE OF CONTENTS

Part III: A New Model of Health Care

Appendices

FOREWORD

It is a strange paradox of modern life that, despite our obsession with curing disease and prolonging life, as a society we still have no framework for achieving true health and maximizing human performance and potential. Even the complementary and alternative medicine approaches that have grown so greatly in use still focus largely on symptom reduction and disease treatment.

Yet, for more than one hundred years, chiropractic has been built on a unique philosophy that recognizes living organisms as possessing a profound, inborn drive toward health and that has as its goal unleashing the body's ability to fully express its inborn potential. The profession as a whole, however, has to date been only partially successful in sharing that profound philosophy clearly and succinctly with other healing professions and the public. The wholesale change in health care approaches that our chiropractic colleges and practitioners envision has yet to become reality—in part, I believe, because we have not yet adequately articulated our philosophy of health.

Although the use and acceptance of chiropractic is at an all-time high, its advancement has been hampered by the lack of published works that clearly espouse the tenets and purposes of the profession and illuminate its far-reaching impact for the lay audience. They say that without the printed word there can be no revolution. Perhaps this thoughtful and balanced work will provide the treatise needed to fuel such a revolution in public thought regarding true health and the contribution chiropractic can make in helping individuals achieve it.

One of the things that impressed me most as I read the book was the comprehensive and straightforward manner in which it is presented. The author clearly has no hidden personal or political agenda he is working to further and so provides a refreshing, candid and complete explanation of the complex chiropractic profession and its practitioners. He explores such key topics as the differences between a mechanistic (traditional medicine) and vitalistic (chiropractic philosophy) approach to health; the history of chiropractic; how the brain and spinal cord work together to coordinate body function; the impact of vertebral subluxation on body function; how to select a doctor of chiropractic and what to expect from chiropractic care. Most important, he accepts readers where they are—from skeptics to devoted patients—and provides them with valuable information that empowers them to make their own decisions regarding their health and health care.

Dr. Lenarz utilizes a no-nonsense approach and real-life case studies the reader can relate to. He answers common questions and addresses frequent misconceptions without preaching or becoming defensive. He covers the specific issues an individual considering chiropractic care might raise, yet consistently brings in the bigger picture of total health maximization. He clearly captures the chiropractic philosophy and lifestyle.

As president of the Palmer Chiropractic Colleges (a system that includes the world's first and largest chiropractic college and the "Fountainhead of Chiropractic"), I am committed to working with individuals such as Dr. Lenarz to bring a health care revolution into being in our lifetimes. Chiropractic has a singular philosophy of human function and health that makes us uniquely positioned and qualified to open, lead and advance public discourse regarding a vitalistic approach to health. It is our responsibility to speak loudly and clearly to the issue. This book does so beautifully.

Guy F. Riekeman, D.C.
President of the Palmer Chiropractic Colleges

INTRODUCTION: SARAH'S STORY

Sedro-Woolley is a small town north of Seattle. It is located near the foot of Mount Baker, a picturesque snowcapped peak that sits in the midst of the North Cascade Mountains. Originally a logging town, in recent years it has become a bedroom community for the larger cities to its west and south. It is a nice-looking place, working hard to keep its small-town feel; its one main downtown street is lined with black cast-iron streetlamps. I practice chiropractic here. My office faces Ferry Street, a tree-lined avenue with Victorian houses for several blocks. In fourteen years of practice I have come to love this town and its people. I also have experienced many miracles.

Sarah was one such "miracle" patient. She was born in a hospital in Spokane, Washington, and her birth was complex and troublesome. After a long, difficult labor, as the baby's head began to appear it was discovered that the umbilical cord was wrapped around her neck—not once but three times. Luckily, the attending doctor was both skilled and inventive. Realizing the danger of the situation, he pushed Sarah back up the birth canal before the cord strangled her. Then he reached inside, cut the umbilical cord free from her neck, and delivered the child.

After the birth, however, there was an unexpected problem: Sarah would stop breathing every time her mother attempted to nurse her. She would not start breathing again until she was artificially resuscitated. This was occurring fifteen to twenty times per day, and doctors couldn't figure out what was causing it. The hospital told Sarah's parents, Tom and Rachel, that they couldn't take their daughter home because her chances for survival without medical intervention seemed doubtful. The baby was also restless and irritable, and never slept more than one or two hours at a time. Six weeks after her birth, Sarah was still confined to the hospital, and her parents were growing desperate.

Rachel's parents, Dave and Eileen, live in Sedro-Woolley. For years they have used chiropractic as part of their family's regular health maintenance. I had taken care of Rachel as she was growing up, but because she had married and moved to the other side of the state, I had not seen her for at least a year. One day Dave came in to see me and told me the story of Sarah and her problem. "I just know there's something you can do for her, Dr. Lenarz," Dave said, his usual confidence in chiropractic augmented by the pride and worry of a new grandfather.

As a father myself, I could only imagine the agonizing experience Rachel and her husband were going through. "I don't know if I can help your granddaughter," I told Dave gently. "But if the birth trauma caused injury to the upper neck, misalignment of bones in this area could be affecting Sarah's ability to breathe."

"Would you go to Spokane to examine her?" Dave asked eagerly. "The hospital won't release her, so you'll have to do it there. It's a short flight, and I'll buy your ticket."

I shook my head. "I doubt the hospital would allow a chiropractor to examine one of their patients," I said. "But I can try. I've gone into nursing homes and hospitals to give adjustments to patients who request it, and I'm willing to do so in this case." Dave left my office, promising to get back to me with more information.

Fortunately, the airplane ride and visit to the hospital were not needed. Two weeks after my conversation with Dave, Rachel and Tom were allowed to take their daughter home for a trial period. The hospital staff attached Sarah to a portable monitor that informed her parents if she stopped breathing, and trained them to resuscitate the child. Instead of going home, however, Rachel, Tom, and Sarah came straight to Sedro-Woolley.

They entered my office late Friday afternoon after a busy day. All the other patients had gone, and my staff was preparing to close up for the night. Sarah nestled in Rachel's arms, but the tranquil picture of mother and child was marred by a network of wires running from somewhere beneath her blanket to a briefcase-sized monitor with lights, buttons, and knobs that Dad was carrying on his shoulder. Sarah was a beautiful little angel—but she also appeared distressed and uncomfortable, with a furrowed brow. My heart began to beat quickly, and I prayed that I could help this child and this family.

I asked Rachel to put her daughter down on the table for a moment. Gently I performed my normal chiropractic pediatric exam on Sarah, running my fingers along the sides of her tiny neck, checking her range of motion by turning her head slowly from side to side. I wanted to determine if there was any misalignment of a spinal bone in the upper neck, which might be causing interference to the nervous system. We took low-dose X rays, and they confirmed my suspicions: There was a large misalignment of Sarah's top neck bone (the atlas), most likely caused by her traumatic birth. The good news was, I knew I could help.

When I work with babies, I use a special device, a kind of portable "table" that I wear around my neck. It allows me to make the fine, very small adjustments babies usually require. As Rachel held Sarah, I stood next to them and placed Sarah's head against the device. Her head was just about at the level of my heart; one of her ears pointed toward my chest. I brought my right hand around to the other side of Sarah's neck (the side facing away from my chest), and with my middle finger I felt for the atlas, the bone I wanted to adjust. There it was—the misplaced bone that was choking off this child's life force. I put my left middle finger on top of the right, and I gave the bone a quick, gentle pull toward my chest. That was it: a movement of no more than a quarter of an inch, and the bone itself probably moved half that.

While the adjustment was minuscule, the transformation in Sarah was enormous. Within seconds Sarah's brow unfurled. The tension in her little face melted away, and she became uncommonly calm. Rachel took her daughter into another room to nurse her—and for the first time in her short and difficult life, Sarah ate without any interference to her breathing. From that point on, Sarah's development was completely normal. I saw her once more, three months later, for a follow-up adjustment, and then sent her and her parents on their way.

A transformation like Sarah's is no small thing, and even though I have been graced to see many lives transformed through chiropractic, I always experience feelings of awe and gratitude when I witness these changes. Just a few examples:

- Shirley was afflicted with debilitating headaches for fifty years. With a course of chiropractic adjustments, she became pain-free for the first time in her life.

- William had extreme low back pain that kept him from driving, sitting, or standing for any period of time. The doctor felt only drugs and surgery would help him, but his wife persuaded him to see me. I found three misaligned vertebrae in his neck and started treating him, and within a few sessions his pain had almost completely disappeared.

- Beverly had severe sciatic nerve pain down her left leg. She was very skeptical when she came to my office and I told her her neck needed to be adjusted; how could a neck adjustment help her leg? But after a couple of weeks, her sciatic pain was completely gone.

- Ron came to me with lower back pain that was so severe he had to crawl from the garden to the house on all fours. Now that he gets regular chiropractic care, his pain is completely gone, and he says he feels young again.

- Dan, an older gentleman with back and leg pain (some of it due to combat injuries from World War II), was amazed by the effects of his sessions. Not only did his back pain and frequent headaches disappear, but he no longer needed the eyeglasses he'd been using for fifty years.

There is magic hidden within all living things. It is the same magic that was released when Sarah was allowed to breathe normally again, when Ron walked normally after one session, when Dan put down his trifocals, and when Shirley had her first headache-free day after a lifetime of agony. This book is about learning to connect with that magic: how to find it, see it, and use it to attain and maintain optimal health.

Like many people, I first came to chiropractic because I was in pain. In 1983 I was twenty-five years old and working as a laborer in a metalworking shop in Pittsburgh. My life experience at that point had been varied, to say the least: After graduating from high school, instead of going to Temple University to study sociology (as my parents wanted me to), I had moved into an ashram in San Antonio, Texas. From there I went through three-plus years of college, a marriage, and a divorce; I started and left a carpet-cleaning business; and finally I found myself with a chronically sore shoulder from pushing a broom at the Kerotest Valve Company.

A friend of mine recommended I see his chiropractor, Dr. Alan Berman, and so I made an appointment. I had a vague notion that a chiropractor was some kind of alternative back pain and joint doctor, but didn't hold out a lot of hope for Dr. Berman's being able to help me. On my very first visit, however, I began to learn the truth about what chiropractic is all about.

"Chiropractors aren't just 'ache and pain, sprain and strain' doctors," Dr. Berman told me. "Chiropractic is about natural healing. It is based on the concept that in every living thing there is an inborn, innate wisdom always striving for health. Chiropractors believe that there is something infinite and perfect in the universe, which forms the very basis of life." In the chiropractor's office I found a healing profession based on an understanding that there is something greater than the rather mechanical approach taken by conventional medicine. Instead, chiropractic recognizes that our bodies are part and parcel of an infinite intelligence that wants to express itself through radiant, natural health.

My spiritual and life experiences had taught me to believe in the existence of something that was far beyond the limits of intellectual understanding, but I never imagined that a healing art and science could embody this truth. Now, at twenty-five, I had finally discovered what I wanted to be when I grew up: a chiropractor. From that first visit my life has never been the same.

Chiropractic works—and it can work for you. Not only can the chiropractic adjustment improve your health whether you have back pain or not, but the principles upon which chiropractic is based will also provide you with a deeper understanding of the true nature of health, disease, and the full expression of life. I have written this book to share this truth with people who are wary or skeptical about chiropractic (until they see and feel its effects in their lives), as well as with those who have found great benefit from chiropractic and want to know how they can support their health in other ways.

I have divided this book's contents into three sections. Part I will share the fundamentals of both chiropractic philosophy and practice. You'll learn about the vast Universal Intelligence that underlies every speck of matter and energy in the cosmos, and how it expresses itself within living beings as Innate Intelligence—the creative, driving force that brings us into existence and sustains our very cells with its power. You'll learn that pain can be the body's signal that the flow of Innate Intelligence is being blocked, and how pain can be both a problem and a gift. You'll discover the fundamental premises of how subluxations—the blocks of Innate Intelligence—occur, and how chiropractic works with the body's own healing mechanisms to restore optimal functioning without drugs or surgery. By the end of Part I, you'll have a thorough understanding of what chiropractic is, why it works, and how valuable its philosophy can be in promoting abundant health and well-being in your life.

In Part II you'll learn how to choose a chiropractor whose style and philosophy suit your own attitudes about health. You'll get helpful hints about what to expect when you go to the chiropractor, what your first visit will be like, and what a course of treatment might consist of. You'll also learn how to adopt what I call the "chiropractic lifestyle": making choices that support greater health, energy, and vitality. We'll talk about the best forms of exercise to support your chiropractic care, what nutritional choices are available to you, and how to reduce stress and increase relaxation. We'll discuss approaching your life and health as a process rather than a goal, one where every choice you make either contributes to or subtracts from your overall experience of vitality. And we'll look at chiropractic care for two very special groups: children and seniors.

Part III helps put chiropractic into the context of the larger picture of health care in America today. We'll talk about the successes and failures of conventional allopathic medicine, and why it's so important for you as a health care consumer to make informed, conscious choices rather than following the crowd. Then we'll explore some questions you can ask and choices you can make as you create your health care plan for life.

Ultimately, this book is all about choices. In today's vast health care marketplace, we are inundated with information about this discovery and that innovation, this study and that warning, advice on everything from which vitamins to take and which exercises to do to how often we should go to the bathroom. Sarah's parents and grandparents were able to make choices that caused a miracle to occur. By reading this book, understanding what I call the "chiropractic way," and following the practices described in its pages, I believe you, too, can choose to create your own miracle of abundant health.

THE CHIROPRACTIC WAY

PART I

The Principles

How Chiropractic Care Can Stop Pain and Help You Regain Your Health

Winifred is a feisty seventy-six-year-old lady with a mischievous smile. She came to my office because she was experiencing chronic back pain and a lack of energy. In the course of my examination, she revealed that she suffered from emphysema, which caused extreme shortness of breath and limited her physical activities. Sleep apnea also caused her to wake up three to five times a night. She was very direct and told me up front that she considered chiropractors "quacks" and the people who swore by them "fruitcakes." (Winifred has never been afraid of speaking her mind.) But she felt conventional medicine offered her only medication, which she had already found unhelpful, and she was afraid of its possible side effects.

I measured Winifred's range of motion, X-rayed her spine and neck, and determined that a course of chiropractic adjustments would help correct certain misalignments in her spine. I recommended a course of treatment consisting of three visits a week the first two weeks and two visits a week the next four weeks, and then we'd see how things were going. Winifred was skeptical—she's a real "show me" lady—but she agreed to give chiropractic a try.

After she noticed significant improvement within a few visits, she told me, "Dr. Lenarz, if I could find some reason other than the chiropractic treatment, I would gladly put the credit elsewhere." But she couldn't ignore the fact that her back pain was gone, her sleep was much improved, and even her emphysema eased significantly. She found she had more energy and stamina. At one visit she bragged that she had taken a ten-hour car trip with no pain or stiffness—and at her age, she said, that was remarkable.

Winifred is typical of many chiropractic patients: They come to the chiropractor as a second, third, or even last resort. Many have tried to handle their conditions with conventional medicine, only to be disappointed with the results. They walk into the chiropractor's office dubiously, not sure whether this new kind of treatment will help, but often desperate for any relief. Like Winifred, they've heard all kinds of bad things about chiropractors: that they're not "real" doctors; that they twist, push, and pull you and cause lots of pain; that the results are temporary at best; and that patients have to keep coming for the rest of their lives to get any real benefit.

With all that bad press, why on earth do people continue to go to chiropractors? And with the forces of conventional medicine arrayed against the practice of chiropractic for most of its hundred-year history, why is chiropractic still the *second-largest health care system* in America and the largest drug-free healing profession in the world? For one very simple and obvious reason: *Chiropractic works.* Every year millions of people use chiropractic to eliminate their pain, and in the process they discover a new approach to health and well-being.

In numerous studies chiropractic has proven to be one of the most effective treatments for back pain, neck pain, headaches, and other musculoskeletal ailments. But at its foundation chiropractic is not really about treatment of pain (although it is very effective at doing so). In chiropractic philosophy, pain relief is really just the side effect of a properly functioning spinal system. Other side effects of chiropractic care include relief from many other conditions and diseases—everything from chronic tonsillitis to high blood pressure to ear problems to digestive ailments and more. Chiropractic treatments help millions of people to live healthier, happier lives, because they restore the body to its proper and natural state.

If you, like Winifred, are skeptical, or if you simply want to know more about chiropractic, I hope this book will show you how you can benefit from incorporating chiropractic into your health care regimen. If you are already going to a chiropractor, you'll learn more about the principles underlying the results you have experienced. Chiropractic is so much more than simply a means of relieving pain; it is a way to a healthier life. Chiropractors believe that health is our natural state and that it can best be maintained through supporting the body in a natural, noninvasive way. Chiropractic philosophy is based on *restoring the body's natural functioning and eliminating obstacles to health* rather than treating symptoms or curing disease.

Strangely enough, it seems that science is finally catching up with what chiropractors have believed all along. The underlying theories of chiropractic as articulated by its founders over a hundred years ago are in line with some of the most cutting-edge research in the field of mind-body medicine. And even though the relationship between conventional medicine and chiropractic is uneasy at best, scientific evidence of the efficacy of chiropractic treatment is mounting every day.

▶ What Is Chiropractic?

If you ask most people what a chiropractor does, their answer will be, "He cracks your back." If you ask what's called a "narrow scope" chiropractor the same question, you'll hear, "A chiropractor reduces subluxations that impede the normal functioning of the spine. Once these subluxations are reduced, normal function can be restored." (You'll learn about subluxations in Chapter 5.) If you ask a "broad scope" chiropractor, you might hear, "We use a variety of techniques that allow the body's natural state of health to express itself fully." And if you ask many conventional medical doctors, you'll hear, "A chiropractor does very little at all, and nothing of any lasting value."

Obviously, I don't subscribe to the last statement, but none of the other statements is a full picture of chiropractic, either. Chiropractic is a science, an art, and a philosophy. It is a science that deals primarily with the spine and central nervous system. Like conventional medicine, it is based upon scientific principles of (1) diagnosis through testing and empirical observation and (2) treatment based upon the practitioner's rigorous training and clinical experience. Unlike conventional medicine, which relies primarily on drugs and/or surgery to heal disease, chiropractic uses manual manipulation, or *adjustments,* of the spine to correct large or small misalignments that have affected the proper flow of communication between the brain, the nervous system, and the rest of the body. Once the spine is realigned to its proper position, the nerves can do their job without impediment, and the patient experiences greater health.

Like conventional medicine, chiropractic is not just a science; it is also an art. Only in the case of chiropractic, it is the art of all things natural. The function of chiropractic is not to heal disease or even to relieve pain, although both of those effects may occur in the course of chiropractic treatment. Ultimately, the goal of the chiropractic art is to *restore the body to its natural state,* which is one of radiant health. In the pursuit of this art, chiropractors work with the body's own energy, guiding bones and tissues that have been damaged through trauma or misuse back to their correct positions. When the bones and soft tissues are returned to their proper states, the vital pathway between the brain and the body is restored. Then the chemical, neurological, and mechanical processes of the body function as they are supposed to.

But perhaps most important, chiropractic is a powerful, rich, and meticulous *philosophy* about the causes of life, health, and disease. Chiropractic believes that inside each of us is an innate wisdom that wants to express itself as perfect health and well-being. Chiropractic's primary focus is simply to remove any physiological blocks to the proper expression of the body's innate wisdom; once those blocks are removed, health is the natural result.

I believe chiropractic philosophy has the potential to cause a worldwide revolution in healing, one that can bring a deeper understanding and create a safer and saner health care industry. But perhaps most important, chiropractic can make a difference in *your* life. It can help you grasp the true nature of health and disease. I know that for my patients and myself, chiropractic helps us to realize that health is a simple, attainable goal. With that knowledge, we can take control of our own health care choices on a completely new level.

▶ A Brief History of an Ancient Practice

Manipulation and/or adjustment of the spine have existed since the beginning of human civilization. An ancient Chinese text indicates that manipulation techniques were being used in that country as early as 2700 B.C.E. In Egypt, a fragment of papyrus dating from 1600 B.C.E. describes a treatment for a dislocated jaw: "Put your two thumbs upon the end of the two rami of the mandible [jawbone] inside his mouth and your fingers under his chin, and you should cause them to fall back so that they rest in their places." Societies all over the ancient world—Babylon, Syria, India, Tibet, Japan; Native American tribes such as the Sioux, Winnebago, and Creek; South American groups of Mayan, Aztec, Toltec, Tarascan, and Zoltec Indians, and the Incas—practiced manipulation as a means of relieving pain and restoring the body to normal function.

Conventional Western medicine, however, traces its roots back to ancient Greece. Over twenty-four hundred years ago, around 400 B.C.E., in the school of the great physician Hippocrates (the legendary father of what we call today "conventional" medicine), students were taught that disease was not a result of supernatural forces or the displeasure of the gods, as had once been believed. Instead, the Hippocratic philosophy was based on the premise that a human body was subject to the same forces and laws as nature itself. Therefore, it was possible for humankind to have a role in the curing of disease and the maintenance of health.

At the school of Hippocrates, the beliefs of conventional medicine and the principles that today underlie chiropractic were one and the same. As described in the Hippocratic text *On the Nature of Man,* a healthy body is one that is "in balance," and illness is the result of an imbalance in one of the body's systems. The job of the Hippocratic physician was to help the body preserve its balance through healthy living, or to restore the balance once it was disturbed through accident or illness. But how? Mostly by relying on the healing power of nature. Instead of focusing on the disease itself, physicians were directed to get the patient healthy primarily through exercise, diet, manipulation, and rest, and then the disease would be eliminated. Another text, *On Ancient Medicine,* states, "Our natures are the physicians of our diseases." Physicians were directed, first, to "do no harm" (a phrase still found in the Hippocratic oath every doctor takes), and second, to ease symptoms to allow the body to heal itself. Because the human body was greatly revered, cutting into it was considered close to sacrilegious. Therefore, physicians had to rely upon observation and natural means to effect a cure.

One of these natural means was manipulation. In the sixty or so works and fragments that constitute our entire knowledge of what was taught at the Hippocratic school, several of them—including *On Fractures, On Setting Joints by Leverage,* and *On the Articulations*—describe contemporary knowledge of the musculoskeletal system and its treatment. "Get knowledge of the spine," says one text, "for this is the requisite for many diseases." These texts explain the difference between complete dislocations (luxations) and partial dislocations (subluxations) of bone. There is also a description of manipulation of a hump on a patient's spine: The patient was to lie facedown on a surface covered with soft material, and the physician then would apply force to the hump using his hand, his foot, or even a board. This would push the bone back into its natural position.

Physicians in ancient Greece, and later in the Roman Empire, drew upon the knowledge and texts of the Hippocratic school to treat disease and preserve health. (Remember, both these societies idolized the athlete as the height of the expression of humankind, so the maintenance of health with diet, exercise, and clean living was promoted—or at least given a lot of lip service.) But with the fall of the Roman Empire and the resulting loss of much of the knowledge of ancient times, medicine retreated to its roots in superstition and ignorance. Western medicine was kept alive by Islamic physicians and dedicated monks in far-flung monasteries, who preserved texts and doggedly continued to observe and treat illness as best they could. But for hundreds of years—even as late as the eighteenth century—the primary treatments prescribed by physicians for illness included purging (with laxatives or emetics), bloodletting (draining the body of excess or "bad" blood), and cupping, where glasses were heated and placed on the body to scald the affected areas and pull the diseased "humors" out of the body.

People who didn't live close to monasteries (or couldn't afford doctors) still got sick, however, and often they turned to folk medicine practitioners for help. Many of these practitioners prescribed a wide variety of efficacious herbal-based remedies to treat illnesses. Another category of "lay doctor" was the bonesetter. Bonesetters didn't just fix broken legs or arms, however; they also were experts in manipulating the spine and other joints. Like most professions, bonesetting was passed from father to son (or daughter—women could be bonesetters, too; one of the most famous bonesetters in eighteenth-century England was Sally Mapp, who did well enough at the profession to be consulted by the gentry for her skills). Even as late as the twentieth century, bonesetters were still practicing their art in small rural villages in Europe.

By the nineteenth century, however, Western medicine had begun more closely to resemble the profession we know today.

Physicians would use their own experience and prior training in medicine to diagnose illness based on their observation of the patient's symptoms. They then would prescribe a combination of drugs, surgery, and (occasionally) lifestyle changes that would alleviate the patient's symptoms and perhaps even cure the underlying condition. But medicine, while becoming more refined as a practice, was still a fairly risky endeavor for the patient. The number of drugs available was small (opiates, such as laudanum, and purgatives being the main categories), and their effects often harsh and imprecise. Surgery was an even more dangerous option, with few remedies for the infection that often set in afterward. For the general population, a visit to the doctor was the last resort rather than the first response to an illness, usually undertaken only after trying every possible folk remedy or patent medicine available. This is not to say that advances in medicine didn't benefit the population as a whole; medical understanding of the nature, causes, and treatment of infectious diseases was an enormous boon to humankind. However, there were still many physical problems nineteenth-century medicine was unable to treat effectively.

Through the years certain physicians had used manipulation of the spine and joints as part of their treatments. Some of them had even studied with bonesetters and adopted their techniques. Every now and then references to the potential effects of spinal and joint misalignment would appear in the medical literature of the day. In 1842, for example, a fellow of the Royal College of Surgeons in England wrote: "Every organ and muscle in the body is dependent more or less upon the spinal nerves. . . . When one vertebra forms a slight exception in the regularity of the spinal line, either by height or distance from its fellows, a serious train of nervous symptoms may supervene."

Then, late in the nineteenth century, two new healing professions based on the ancient practice of manipulation appeared in the American Midwest. The first of these was osteopathy. Andrew Taylor Sill, a bonesetter from Missouri, had served as a surgeon and soldier during the Civil War and had come away dissatisfied with the limited ability of surgery and drugs to help his suffering patients. He wanted to find a way to tap into the body's natural healing abilities, and turned to manipulation of the bones and joints. Sill discovered that when joints and bones were manipulated (moved into their proper position and alignment), the results included increased circulation and greater health in the patient. A whole range of conditions such as digestive problems, low energy, specific and nonspecific pain, and so on would ease or disappear altogether. In 1874 Sill published his discoveries, and called this new profession osteopathy (*osteo* is the Greek word for bone). He traveled throughout the Midwest teaching his techniques, and eventually founded a school of osteopathic medicine in Missouri, which granted its first doctor of osteopathy (D.O.) degree in 1892.

▶ The Founding of Chiropractic

During the same years that Andrew Sill was investigating the effect of joint manipulation on health, another man was examining the power of manipulation on one specific area: the spine. D. D. (David Daniel) Palmer had studied the then-popular method of magnetic healing (what we would probably call today "healing touch") and was also familiar with the principles of manipulation, either through hearing of Sill's work or perhaps by studying with a bone-setter himself. But he was still curious as to the causes of disease. "What difference was there in the two persons that caused one to have pneumonia . . . typhoid or rheumatism, while his partner, similarly situated, escaped?" he asked. Palmer theorized that many conditions of ill health were due not to general joint problems but to misaligned vertebrae in the spine, which interfered with the nerve signals sent from the brain through the spinal cord to the rest of the body.

In 1895 Palmer's theories were put to the test. Harvey Lillard, a janitor in Palmer's office building in Davenport, Iowa, had been deaf for seventeen years. The man told Palmer he had exerted himself while stooping, felt something give way in his back, and his hearing had disappeared. Palmer examined him and discovered that one of the man's vertebrae was severely out of alignment. He persuaded the janitor to lie facedown on a couch and, using his hand, pushed the vertebra back into its proper position. "Soon," Palmer reported, "the man could hear as before." D. D. Palmer continued to treat patients with different conditions using spinal manipulation, and he saw significant results with many of them. He termed this new approach to healing *chiropractic,* from the Greek word *cheri,* "hand," and *praktikos,* "practice." (Interestingly enough, the words *surgery* and *surgeon* derive from the same Greek root, *cheri,* denoting the use of the hands in their work.)

Over the next several years, D. D. Palmer combined his experiences with patients at his clinic, further research into anatomy and physiology, and his background in magnetic or energetic healing, and created the foundations of what the world now knows as chiropractic. The premises were simple:

- Over time, due to either a trauma or a repeated abnormal movement, small misalignments can occur in the bones of the spine (the vertebrae).

- These misalignments can interfere with the flow of nerve impulses/energy/information from the brain through the spinal cord and nerves to the body.

- When nerve impulses are impeded or blocked, the body can no longer function in the way it was designed, and the results can include pain, limited motion, and a range of symptoms and diseases that, on the surface, may seem unrelated to the spine or nerves.

- Using precise manual manipulation of the spine, chiropractors bring the patient's vertebrae back into alignment.

- When this is done, normal nerve function is restored, and the body can once again function fully, in the way it was intended, resulting in alleviation of symptoms and greater health.

D. D. Palmer also posited that there is an intelligence within the human body that is a microcosm or manifestation of the greater intelligent energy that forms, supports, and exists in every part of the universe. The brain and nerves are some of the primary conduits of this energy in the body. Thus, when vertebral misalignments, or subluxations, are corrected by a chiropractor's manipulation, the life force can flow throughout the body as it was designed to, and we experience our natural state of radiant health and well-being. (While Palmer's belief in the life force was questioned for years, recent studies in fields such as psychoneuroimmunology and psychobiology are showing the effects of mind upon matter, and how interference with messages from the brain and nerves to the rest of the body can indeed contribute to a wide variety of conditions and diseases.)

Since the early years of the twentieth century, chiropractic has continued to grow as a profession and a discipline. Fostered by D. D. Palmer's son, B. J. Palmer, chiropractic schools were established in several states and cities. As the profession became established, chiropractors built on D. D. Palmer's original techniques to create a range of different kinds of treatment options for patients. (I'll talk about these in Chapter 6.) Eighteen accredited schools in the United States and Canada and nine schools in other countries now offer degrees in chiropractic medicine, and all fifty states have licensing and qualifying processes for those who wish to practice chiropractic. Today there are approximately sixty-five thousand chiropractors practicing in the United States and another twenty thousand in other countries. In a little over a century, chiropractic has grown to become the second largest health care system in the United States, and the largest drug-free health profession in the world.

▶ Myths About Chiropractic

As successful as chiropractic has become, there are a lot of myths about chiropractic floating around in the general public—as my patient Winifred demonstrated. Some of these myths are a result

of chiropractic's differences with the conventional medical establishment (see Part III), and some arise from misunderstandings of
the basic philosophies of chiropractic. Just as I did with Winifred,
I'd like to address a few of these myths right up front.

- **Chiropractors are not real doctors.** As I mentioned earlier,
chiropractors are medical professionals licensed in every U.S.
state, as well as the District of Columbia, Puerto Rico, and the
U.S. Virgin Islands. Today most chiropractic schools require a
minimum of two years of undergraduate study, with emphasis on the basic sciences, for a student to be considered for
admission. According to statistics gathered by Terry A. Rondberg, D.C. (president of the World Chiropractic Alliance and
founder of *The Chiropractic Journal*), the typical chiropractic cur-
riculum is four years long and includes over 2,885 hours of
instruction in anatomy, physiology, pathology, chemistry,
microbiology, neurology, diagnosis, radiology, orthopedics,
even psychiatry and obstetrics. Fields such as geriatrics and
pediatrics are also part of the chiropractic student's training.

As part of their education, chiropractic students also complete approximately nine hundred hours of work in a clinical
setting, assisting licensed chiropractors, observing, and learning. There is additional training in nutrition, palpation, and
different adjusting techniques, all under the supervision of
working doctors of chiropractic. Once students earn their
doctor of chiropractic (D.C.) degree, they must then pass the
state licensing exam for the location where they wish to practice, as well as a practical exam and interview by the state
board. Virtually all students also take the National Board
of Chiropractic Examination, which is a comprehensive test
accepted by most states as a licensing exam. Once a chiropractor has passed these tests, he or she can open a practice.

As you can see, chiropractors receive extensive, scientifi
cally based training combined with many hours of practical
work. Just like conventional medical doctors, they are medical professionals subject to testing, examination, licensing,

and monitoring by state and national peer-review boards. Chiropractic is also recognized as a valid part of the overall health care system: Federal and state programs such as Medicare, Medicaid, and state workers' compensation programs cover chiropractic, and all federal agencies accept sick-leave certificates signed by doctors of chiropractic. Chiropractic care is covered in the health insurance policies of over 75 percent of the insurance carriers in the United States. Many plans also will allow patients to have a doctor of chiropractic as their primary-care physician.

• **Chiropractors push and pull and twist you, and the treatments hurt.** The usual response to chiropractic adjustment is "Is that it?" Most adjustments are quick, painless, and fairly minor. It doesn't take a lot of movement for a vertebra to slip back into place, yet the difference between a misaligned bone and one that's properly aligned is huge. Even in some of the more dramatic kinds of adjustments (where the chiropractor has the patient twist his hips one way and shoulders another, then uses this twist to help lever the vertebra back into place), the usual experience is relief of pain rather than more discomfort. Some patients can experience a little soreness for a day or so after a session, but that's usually caused by muscles that have been functioning improperly for a long time having to adapt to functioning correctly. You'll learn more about how an adjustment works in Chapter 5.

According to many surveys, patients are actually far more satisfied with their chiropractic treatment than they are with conventional medical care. I believe one of the reasons for this is that many patients feel much better immediately after their sessions. How many patients can say that after visiting their conventional medical doctor?

• **You have to keep going for the rest of your life to achieve any benefit.** Many patients come to chiropractic because they are in pain, and once the pain is gone, they stop going to the chiropractor. And that's fine—if all they want is relief from pain. But remember, chiropractic philosophy is based on allowing the body to achieve and maintain its natural state of radiant health and well-being, and to do that, we need to take care of our spines on a regular basis.

I hold patient education talks in my practice every week, and in them I ask, "How many of you have heard that once you go to a chiropractor, you always have to go?" (There are usually several sheepish grins and half-raised hands at this point.) I continue, "It's just like those darn dentists. Once you start going, they expect you to come in for a cleaning every six months!"

Dentists today practice preventive medicine. You go in every six months and get a cleaning and a checkup. The dentist examines your teeth for normal wear and tear, catches small problems (like cavities, gum disease, and so on), and fixes them while they're minor. However, if you don't go to the dentist until you're in pain, you run the risk of needing far more extensive, painful, and costly work (like root canals, periodontal work, tooth extractions, bridgework, even dentures).

Just like your teeth, your spine experiences normal wear and tear—you walk, drive, sit, stand, and move every day, sometimes in ways that create misalignment and even discomfort. When you see your chiropractor once a month, or once every three months, for what we call "maintenance care," then he or she can catch and handle any small problems quickly and easily. But if you wait until you're in pain, then it will take the chiropractor longer, and you'll need more treatments than you would have if you'd been coming in for regular care.

There are two exceptions to equating regular dental and chiropractic care. First, most chiropractic visits are a lot more enjoyable than most trips to the dentist. And second, while I have great respect for dentists (and value my own teeth highly), I believe that keeping your spine healthy is more important even than keeping your teeth sound. After all, if you have problems with your teeth, as a last resort the dentist can give you a set of dentures to replace them, but there is no equivalent replacement for your spine. Regular chiropractic care can help you feel better, move with more freedom, and stay healthier throughout your lifetime. To me, that's worth a half an hour every three months.

- **Only New Age people use chiropractors.**   If it's true that only New Agers use chiropractic, then I guess most professional athletes in the United States fit into that category, because the roster of sports stars that use chiropractic is impressive. To list just a few of the most well known: Michael Jordan, Charles Barkley, and Scottie Pippen from basketball; Mark McGwire and Brett Butler from baseball; Tiger Woods from golf; Joe Montana, Ricky Bell, and Emmett Smith from football (as well as entire teams, including the Atlanta Falcons, San Francisco 49ers, Detroit Lions, Denver Broncos, and Dallas Cowboys); Wayne Gretzky and Brett Hull from hockey; Olympic athletes Dan O'Brien, Joe Greene, and Mary Lou Retton; tennis greats John McEnroe and Jimmy Connors; bodybuilder and actor Arnold Schwarzenegger; and scores of others.

I could continue to list people who have benefited from regular chiropractic care, including prominent public figures such as Richard Pryor, Bob Hope, Dixie Carter, Mel Gibson, Robin Williams, Madonna, Denzel Washington, Peter Frampton, David Spade, and Diana, princess of Wales. But what's more important are the twenty-five million Americans just like you who will visit chiropractors every year. If you ask a few of the people you know, I'll bet at least one of them has visited a chiropractor, or knows someone who has. I hope you'll begin to see that chiropractic can provide a valid, valuable, drug-free, natural option when it comes to caring for your health.

Chiropractic is a time-proven, tested means of supporting your continued health and well-being. Doctors of chiropractic are trained, dedicated individuals who provide a specific kind of care that's drug-free, painless, and natural. Millions of people use chiropractic as part of their ongoing health care, to ease or eliminate pain and restore the body to its natural level of optimal functioning. And more and more, individuals are choosing to embrace what I like to call the "chiropractic way" to attain greater health.

▶ The Chiropractic Way

It seems to me that over the course of the twentieth century most Americans lost control over their own health. Sure, there have been enormous advances in conventional medicine and technology, and in circumstances such as traumatic accidents, heart attacks, or other such disasters there is nothing like a top-flight emergency room. But the conventional medical establishment appears to be focused on *curing disease* rather than *gaining health*. Billions of dollars and hundreds of millions of man-hours are spent creating more drugs and finding better surgical techniques and tools. Don't get me wrong, curing disease is a noble goal—but in the process, it seems the idea of maintaining health has been left by the wayside.

I believe that's one of the reasons for the upsurge in interest in what's called alternative medicine. People don't just want to be cured when they're sick; they want to feel *healthy* on a regular basis. Like Winifred, many individuals have tried conventional medicine and been dissatisfied with the results. They have taken medication and suffered with the side effects. They have undergone the pain and trauma of surgery and the tedium of recovery and rehabilitation that follows. They are seeking an alternative way of achieving and maintaining health, one that uses the body's own forces to heal.

More and more, people realize that the lifestyle choices they make daily—what to eat, whether and/or how to exercise, which supplements to take, how they handle stress, even the thoughts they think and the beliefs they hold—are the real keys to health. They're ready to take charge of their own physical well-being, and they're looking for health care providers who will help them in doing so. If you are one of those people, you are not alone. In 1997 the number of visits to alternative medical providers (chiropractors, acupuncturists, naturopaths, homeopaths, etc.) in the United States outnumbered visits to conventional medical doctors for the first time. Every single year since then, the trend has continued to favor alternative medicine. And of all alternative medical treatments, chiropractic is the most popular. It has been and will continue to be in the forefront of this new wave of health. I believe this is due not only to the efficacy of chiropractic treatments but also to the truth and power of chiropractic philosophy.

The chiropractic way is based upon the recognition that health is our natural state, and our main job is simply to eliminate anything that gets in the way of the natural expression of the life force within us. The chiropractic way acknowledges our link to the intelligence and energy that pervade the universe, which formed the first stars and is present in each and every cell. The chiropractic way states that we are in charge of creating our own health and well-being; our health care providers can assist us, but they cannot do it for us. The chiropractic way respects the role of both patient and provider in the creation of health. And finally, the chiropractic way shows us that health is actually a simple and attainable goal once we follow a few basic, commonsense guidelines.

The great philosopher John Locke wrote, "A sound mind in a sound body, is a short but full description of a happy state in this world. He that has these two has little more to wish for; and he that wants either of them will be little the better for anything else." The chiropractic way can help you attain and maintain that happy state of health, which is, indeed, the greatest wealth we have.

2

The Energy of Life:
Your Connection to the Universe

What is life? Where does it come from? What is this wondrous thing we call a human being? And how do the fundamental molecules that make up a strand of DNA "know" how to come together to create living, breathing, conscious creatures—us?

These questions about the origin of life are basic to our very nature. They have intrigued and perplexed scientists, philosophers, and theologians ever since those disciplines first appeared. From the ancient written records of all societies, including the works of Hippocrates and Plato, the Hebrew Bible, the ancient Sanskrit texts of India, and many others, you'll find one thing in common: a recognition that life is mysterious. Life's origin and destination can be theorized about but never proven. Modern science has the ability to measure everything, from the path of the smallest sub-atomic particle over the course of one ten-billionth of a second to the movement of galaxies in the vast untrackable distances of the universe. But as any scientist will acknowledge, life cannot be reduced to the movement of subatomic particles, and conscious-ness cannot be discovered by knowing the electrochemical reac-tions in the brain.

Answering the question "What is life?" is a key component of chiropractic philosophy and has a direct bearing on how chiro-practic works. Surprisingly, theories proposed by some of our most cutting-edge scientific and medical disciplines are coming ever closer to the truths that chiropractic has espoused from the beginning. From astronomy to quantum physics, from neurobiol-ogy to psychoneuroimmunology—chiropractic truths dealing with the source of our own life, and our link to life as it exists all around us, are being discovered by these other disciplines. They explain how our bodies know how to heal themselves, and how we are part and parcel of the energy that imbues every particle of the universe. When you understand the foundations of chiropractic's answer to the question "What is life?" you will see how this partic-ular form of health care can help you express your own life on a more vibrant level.

▶ From Quarks to Quasars: The Energy of the Universe

Astronomer Carl Sagan referred to human beings as "children of the stars." He based this declaration on the theory that all planets (including the earth) and everything on them were created from elements that exist as the result of the formation and dissolution of stars. But how are we related to the universe—or, more impor-tant, how is the universe related to us?

One of the primary tenets of physics today is that ultimately all matter is composed of the same "stuff." Most of us have been taught that everything is made of atoms. We now know that atoms are made of even smaller components called subatomic particles. Subatomic particles form relationships called atoms. (I say "relationships" because subatomic particles can enter and leave atoms at will, being replaced by other subatomic particles performing their same functions.) We have learned that an atom is not a thing but a fluid relationship of particles. Atoms form relationships called molecules, molecules make up relationships called cells, and so on.

The same subatomic particles that make up atoms also express themselves in the form of energy. Ever since Albert Einstein stood theoretical physics on its ear in 1905 with his equation $E=mc^2$, scientists have been exploring the amazing concept that matter and energy are the same stuff. Matter is nothing but an expression of energy in a different form, and energy is matter accelerated to the speed of light. But what is this "stuff" that composes both matter and energy? Where did it come from? And how does it show up in so many different forms? Like the origins of life, the origins of energy and matter have flummoxed scientists throughout history.

But philosophy has stepped in where science faces its limits. One way that philosophy works is by looking at how energy/matter expresses itself. It looks at the galaxies, stars, and planets; at the cohesiveness of an atom; at the interaction of sunlight and cells in green plants; at the millions of ways energy and matter come together. And philosophy says this is not random. There is order and organization to the expression of matter and energy, more than can be explained logically by random happenstance. Order and organization imply that something is doing the organizing, that there is an intelligence underlying the orderly expression of matter and energy. There must be some kind of *Universal Intelligence* that creates and sustains all matter and energy in existence. This particular school of philosophical thought is called *vitalism* (from the Latin root *vita,* "life"), and it is one of the key principles of chiropractic.

By "Universal Intelligence," I don't necessarily mean God in a religious sense, although it does not exclude the possibility that Universal Intelligence is what many people mean when they talk about God. Universal Intelligence is definitely outside of and greater than the parameters of the physical nature of the universe. Because of this, it is ultimately immeasurable by science. Yet, interestingly enough, science has come to recognize the existence of Universal Intelligence, simply because so many phenomena can be explained only by its presence. In his groundbreaking book *Quantum Healing: Exploring the Frontiers of Mind/Body Medicine,* Dr. Deepak Chopra described how quantum physics has moved science toward the recognition of a universal organizing principle in the universe. The solar system, life on earth, the moon pulling on the oceans, and the beating of our hearts are all examples of the brilliant organization of energy and matter. Once we acknowledge this underlying order, *not* believing in Universal Intelligence is actually more absurd than believing in it. It's like believing a house can build itself, or a car can move down a road, make turns, stop, and arrive safely at a destination without someone at the controls. As Chopra puts it, "Science tends to be skeptical in the face of any claim that intelligence is at work in nature. . . . However, if there is nothing outside ordinary reality to hold things and events together, then one is led to a set of impossibilities."

There's a joke about two old friends, a preacher and an atheist. For twenty years these two men have argued back and forth about the existence of intelligence and purpose behind the creation of the universe. One day the preacher has an idea. He goes down into his basement and constructs an elaborate model of the solar system to scale. He builds it so the sun will revolve and the planets will turn in their correct orbits at absolutely accurate speeds. Then he invites his atheist friend over and brings him down into the basement. The atheist is amazed. He looks at the model and says, "Wow, this is incredible! It's one of the most awesome things I've ever seen. Who built it?" And the preacher smiles and replies, "Nobody."

The "happy accident" theory of matter and energy is losing credence, even with scientists. The smaller our investigations into matter and energy and the larger our explorations of the cosmos, the clearer it becomes that some intelligence is creating order out of chaos. (Even chaos has intelligence behind it, as exhibited by chaos theory, a field built around the study of randomness, which has discovered patterns in the most disorganized-seeming responses of matter and energy.) And nowhere is the functioning of Universal Intelligence more evident than in the unique, inexplicable, dynamic interaction of matter and energy we call life.

▶ Innate Intelligence Is the Lifeblood of Life

When manifesting as life, Universal Intelligence has some very specific and unique properties: change, growth, adaptation, and also decay and death. To distinguish between the broad field of Universal Intelligence and its unique expression called life, chiropractic philosophy uses a different term, calling the life force *Innate Intelligence*. Innate Intelligence links life to something far greater than itself, to the energy that formed the first stars and existed before them. It is the ultimate source of energy that powers every living thing, from a single-celled organism to the most complex beings. Innate Intelligence is what teaches DNA to create life from simple strands of carbon molecules and tells plants how to use the energy of the sun to create living cells from carbon dioxide and water. And, as we'll see in Chapter 3, Innate Intelligence runs every single process in the human body without our ever having to think about it.

Science has a hard time with the concept of an intelligence underlying life. With its experiments and proofs and reductions of life to electrochemical reactions, science can appear to be trying to prove life right out of existence. But as anyone who has been present at a death will tell you, there is an enormous contrast between a living body and a dead one. The electrochemical and biological processes are only infinitesimally different in the moments before and after death, but in that infinitesimal change is all the difference in the world. Innate Intelligence is the origin and director of all the processes and systems that science is so good at measuring, but it is beyond any measurements itself. As Einstein and other quantum physicists have said about their own discipline, it's like trying to measure the fourth dimension using three-dimensional equations.

Science is based on inductive reasoning, which works something like this: If we keep breaking down a thing into its smallest components, we will discover its true nature. Inductive reasoning is based on the belief that the sum of the parts is equal to the whole. For instance, if we study and understand how a liver cell works, this helps us to understand how the liver functions. This process certainly has validity—to a point. But where does life arise in this reduction of a human being to the smallest components? Are our subatomic particles alive in the same sense that a human being experiences life? We cannot know. But we do know that we cannot completely define ourselves through the chemistry and physics of our body. We know *we* are something much more.

Science (induction) helps us to understand *how* things work. Philosophy, which is deductive, looks at *why* things are the way they are. Philosophy is based on the idea that the whole is greater than the sum of its parts. One of my favorite examples of the difference between inductive (scientific) and deductive (philosophical) reasoning is the story of two masons at a construction site. Each worker takes one brick at a time and, using a mortar trowel to scoop up and smooth the cement, places a brick at the top of the wall they are building. Each one then cleans off the excess cement with the same trowel, creating a neat and level addition of one more brick to the project. A curious bystander approaches the first mason and asks, "What are you doing?" The mason replies, exasperated, "Can't you see? I'm putting bricks in place to build this wall." The man then goes to the second mason and asks, "What are you doing?" The second mason answers with a smile, "Can't you see? I'm building a magnificent cathedral!"

Both answers are true and accurate; the difference is in the perspective. The placement of the bricks, the smallest component, does not give an accurate description or understanding of the whole. The brick is the *how* of things (induction); the cathedral is the *why* (deduction). In the same way understanding the brick doesn't describe the cathedral, understanding how the cell or the subatomic particle functions does not necessarily explain the why of life. There is something magical, something beyond the how of things, that science can never measure. This immeasurable thing is Innate Intelligence. Though we might be able to reason its possibility or explain it through quantum physics, it is only through the very real experience of this magic in our lives that we can come to know the true motivating force of our very being.

▶ The Cellular Biology of Innate Intelligence

Often it is not just the individual scientific research results that are important but also the ability to maintain an overview of related knowledge, tie together component and disparate bits of information, and create a true understanding of the whole. As in the example of the bricklayers—where one mason is just putting bricks in place while the other is building a cathedral—modern science, and specifically, modern medicine, needs scientists who can see the whole cathedral of life while working with the individual bricks of the body's cells and systems.

Dr. Bruce Lipton is the type of scientist that can see the whole cathedral. Dr. Lipton has a Ph.D. in cellular biology. He is a former Associate Professor of Anatomy at Wisconsin's School of Medicine (1973–1982) and Research Fellow at Stanford University's School of Medicine (1987–1992). Currently he is a visiting professor at Palmer College of Chiropractic in Davenport, Iowa. (The information in this section is based largely on Dr. Lipton's work.) Dr. Lipton states that there has been a recent renaissance in cellular biology that provides insight into the mechanisms underlying energy medicine and the mind-body connection. When this work is fully understood by the larger scientific community, it will show that chiropractors have been correct in their theories for one hundred years and that allopathic medicine in large part is founded on erroneous assumptions. These findings are as earthshaking to the fields of biology and medicine as Einstein's relativity theory was to the old Newtonian view of the universe. Indeed, one of the fundamental problems with allopathic medicine is its basis in Newtonian instead of quantum physics. Quantum physics teaches us that the basis of all matter is not mechanical but energetic. Modern allopathic medicine is still based upon Newtonian physics, explaining the world in terms of mechanical structures and not taking energy into consideration as part of the formula.

Let me give you an example. One of the fundamental beliefs of modern biology and of modern medicine is that *genes control biology.* This belief is called the "Central Dogma" of modern biology. (Interesting how "dogma" is a religious term.) But to understand how this dogma is untrue, we first must trace its origins and then show how modern cellular biology has disproved this critical assumption.

In 1859 Charles Darwin's book, *The Origin of Species,* was published, and from this point on we began to understand that something was passed from parent to child that determined what or who we are. Nearly one hundred years later, in 1953, James Watson and Francis Crick published their groundbreaking research regarding the discovery of DNA—the mechanism of transferring genetic material from parent to offspring. Since 1953, research into this genetic material has continued, and in June 2000 scientists associated with the Human Genome Project and Celera Genomics Corporation announced they had mapped the entire human genetic blueprint. In large part, the impetus for this discovery was the medical model, which says that human beings are biochemical mechanisms controlled by our genes. This genetic determinism posits that who we are physically (and mentally in many instances as well) is determined solely by our genetic makeup. In essence, we are victims of our genes.

But there are some interesting if little-known side issues created by the Human Genome Project and the Central Dogma that underlies it. Genes are made up of DNA, and DNA is a strand of molecules that are used to create proteins. Living things are given all of their characteristics from the proteins created by our DNA. According to the Central Dogma, these proteins determine the shape of our nose, the color of our eyes, and our blood type. Proteins determine the pitch of our voice and the color of our skin. Proteins control all of our physiological functions. All of our physical and many of our basic mental characteristics are the result of different types of protein molecules. DNA sits inside of the nucleus of every cell in the body, and this DNA contains within it the blueprint for all these proteins.

Another type of molecule, RNA, which is a carbon copy of the DNA molecule, conveys messages from the DNA inside of the nucleus to the rest of the cell. Here is a visual representation of the process.

DNA ➡ RNA ➡ Protein
(Physical characteristic or function)

There are approximately 100,000 proteins in the human body. The original understanding among genetic biologists was that each protein has a gene responsible for creating it. Based on this model, they theorized that there must be at least 100,000 genes in the human genome sequence. However, genes create proteins only when and where their specific proteins are needed. Therefore, there has to be some kind of control mechanism, a switch that turns the DNA protein factory on and off. Scientists figured there would have to be about 40,000 additional proteins to adequately control gene function, so it was logical to assume there must be about 140,000 genes in the entire human genome. But then came the announcement that the entire human genome had been mapped—and it contained only 34,000 genes! The geneticists got caught with their "genes" down, so to speak, and in the quest to understand life we were almost back to square one. Whatever controls the genes is at the basis of life; but if genes don't control the vast number of proteins and protein controllers that make up a functioning human body, what does?

Scientists long thought that, much as the human brain controls and coordinates function within the body, the nucleus does the same for the cell. However, recent research has shown this is not true. If you remove the brain from the body, the body ceases to function almost immediately; but if you remove the nucleus from the cell, the cell will continue to function normally for up to *two months.* It was by studying this phenomenon that cellular biologists began to unravel the mystery of the missing control genes. Control was not coming from the DNA and genes in the nucleus: Control of cellular functions came from the membrane of the cell—its "skin"! But rather than the membrane functioning independently, changes in cellular function were created when receptors on the surface of the membrane interacted with signals from the environment. In other words, the control of cellular activity came from the environment! Cellular control doesn't come from our genes; it comes from environmental signals. This new understanding is shown in the model below.

Environ- ➡ Membrane ➡ Signal ➡ DNA ➡ RNA ➡ Protein
mental   from   (Physical
Signal   membrane   characteristic
                                                    or function)

There has long been a debate in biology as to whether we are products of our genetic nature or our environment. These recent breakthroughs in cellular biology tip the scales strongly in favor of the environmental side of the discussion. Genes contain the blueprint for the construction of the proteins, but that's all—just the blueprint. And a blueprint can't build itself; to create what's in the blueprint takes contractors and workers. Genes control nothing. The cell membrane, the receptors on the membrane, the environmental signals, and the proteins within the cell are the contractors and workers that build what the genes can only indicate. The significance of this shift in our fundamental understanding of the life of our cells points to a number of underlying principles that undermine allopathic medical assumptions and support chiropractic philosophy.

Let's look at the medical assumptions first. Traditional allopathic medicine is in large part based upon a centuries-old scientific belief originally expressed by Francis Bacon: that the purpose of science is to learn how to control nature. The enormous scientific energy that went into discovering the human genome was for the purpose of controlling nature. The assumption is that if nature can't do genetics correctly, then humans in all their educated wisdom will learn how to control nature through genetics. This approach treats life like a biochemical machine (Newtonian physics again) in which we can simply take out broken "parts," i.e., genes, and replace them with new ones created in the laboratory. (In fact, much of the private funding for genetic research came from pharmaceutical companies that are now patenting human genes as if they own them.) But as we have seen in far too many cases, science's attempts to control nature produces very serious side effects. For instance, gene therapy, which was promoted with great hope and great fanfare as the cure to all ills, continues to produce far more problems than cures. I am not saying that research into genetics and use of that information for the good of humanity is wrong, but, as you will see in Chapter 14, there are some fundamental problems in the current medical model that arise from the erroneous views of life as biomechanical, and science as the great controller of nature.

But what if we made other assumptions? First, that the purpose of science is to work in harmony with nature, not to control it. Second, that we do not live in a Newtonian world controlled by mechanics, where we can simply remove and replace parts. Instead, we live in a universe that is a continuous, infinite field of intelligent energy. While chiropractic has espoused these principles for over one hundred years, some researchers and physicians within the current medical system are also beginning to understand this new information. These scientists are producing remarkable evidence that explains why chiropractic has been so powerful in its ability to make a difference with a wide variety of health problems.

The underlying assumptions of chiropractic philosophy match perfectly with the newest discoveries of cellular biology and quantum physics. First, chiropractic is based on an understanding that Universal Intelligence (energy) underlies all nature, and it is the continuous interplay between the energy outside of our body (the environment/Universal Intelligence) and the energy inside our body (physiology/Innate Intelligence) that is the basis of life. In addition, the discovery that the control of genes is primarily environmental also correlates with the view of the importance of the nervous system that forms the basis of chiropractic. Each cell is a microcosm of the body. Like the body, each individual cell performs all of the basic functions of life: It eats, digests, eliminates, respires (breathes), reproduces, and metabolizes. Each cell has within it microscopic "organs" called organelles, which carry out specific functions just like our body's organs do. Indeed, it would seem that the functions of these organelles are closely tied to the efficient operation of their larger "cousins." For example, the cells that make up the human digestive system are exceptionally rich in the organelles that cells use to digest. Our body's detoxification organ, the liver, is made up of cells that are exceedingly rich in organelles that aid in cellular detoxification. All of our physiological functions are based on the body's cellular activities.

If, as was explained earlier, the cell membrane relates the cell to its environment, what relates a multicellular organism like a human being to its environment? Primarily the skin, obviously— but also the nervous system. The correlation between the membrane of the cell and the nervous system is further supported by embryology, or the study of human development from fertilized egg to fully-formed child. There are three layers of cells that appear at the very beginning of embryonic development: the ectoderm, the mesoderm, and the endoderm. As the embryo continues to develop, each one of these layers gives rise to very specific types of tissue. The outside layer—the ectoderm—is much like the membrane of a single cell organism. As it develops, the ecto-derm gives rise to both the skin and the nervous system: the tissues that are our interface with the environment.

The nervous system is composed of many components. Our senses are all part of our nervous system; our sense of touch, hot, cold, vision, hearing, taste, and smell are all part of nervous system function. There are also myriad activities that are part of the auto-nomic nervous system, which controls and coordinates our inter-nal environment. From the surface of our body to the innermost aspects of our physiological function, the nervous system creates an unbroken chain of communication and interaction that is at the very core of the cause of life. And because chiropractic adjust-ments remove interference to nervous system function, this form of treatment can be of enormous benefit, not just to the health of the spine but also to the very foundations of human life.

This is just a sampling of the groundbreaking information Dr. Bruce Lipton presents at seminars throughout North America. The research that he has done and the information that he has brought together deepen our understanding of the foundation of life. Over one hundred years ago D. D. Palmer and his son B. J. laid the groundwork in Western society for our current understand-ing. With the work of thousands of chiropractors, and people like Deepak Chopra and Bruce Lipton, the current renaissance in mind-body healing continues.

▶ The Experience of Awe: Our Truest Response to Life

I read an article recently about a couple of scientists who were interested in why human beings all over the world seem to have some belief in a higher power. Psychiatrist Eugene d'Aquili theo-rized that there was something hardwired in humanity's brain that predisposes us to an experience that we call "God" or "mysti-cism" or a more personalized term for this sense of something greater than ourselves. So in the 1990s Andrew Newberg, a radiologist, decided to see if he could prove d'Aquili right. As reported in their book *Why God Won't Go Away: Brain Science and the Biology of Belief,* Newberg and d'Aquili took scans of the level of brain activity in Buddhist monks and Franciscan nuns who were in deep meditation and prayer. Newberg discovered that there were unique patterns of activity in certain areas of the brain when the subjects described themselves as having an experience of oneness with God or the universe.

All very well and good—but are Newberg's scans a true measure of the *experience* of these meditators? If we could have taken scans of Shakespeare's brain when he was writing *Romeo and Juliet,* or Mozart's brain when he composed *Don Giovanni,* or Einstein's brain when he developed the theory of relativity, would we have understood their genius any more than we do by experiencing the play, the opera, or the idea? And if somehow we could make our brains duplicate the exact same patterns that Shakespeare exhibited, would we, too, be able to write plays that will live for hundreds of years? No. There is something about life that eludes measurement, that is subtler than the smallest fragment of energy, the tiniest movement of a neuropeptide molecule, the most fleeting thought. This is the realm of Innate Intelligence—the all-important life energy on which chiropractic is based.

I mentioned in Chapter 1 that B. J. Palmer, the son of chiropractic's founder, D. D. Palmer, took his father's work and turned it into a thriving, philosophically based, scientifically trained discipline now practiced by healing professionals all over the world. But B. J. Palmer was much more than an ambassador of chiropractic. He was a philosopher, a researcher, an entrepreneur, a theorist whose writings anticipated many of the scientific discoveries of the twentieth century. At almost the same time as Albert Einstein was exploring the theory of relativity and quantum physics, and medical researchers were just beginning to understand the chemical and electrical processes that create the biology of the human body, B. J. Palmer was writing about how life and energy are linked together—writing not in dry, academic terms, but in words a poet might use.

We chiropractors work with the subtle substance of the soul. We release the prisoned impulses, a tiny rivulet of force that emanates from the mind and flows over the nerves to the cells and stirs them to life. We deal with the magic power that transforms common food into living, loving, thinking clay; that robes the earth with beauty, and hues and scents the flowers with the glory of the air.

In the dim, dark distant long ago, when the sun first bowed to the morning star, this power spoke and there was life, it quickened the slime of the sea and the dust of the earth and drove the cell to union with its fellows in countless living forms. Through eons of time it finned the fish and winged the bird and fanged the beast. Endlessly it worked, evolving its forms until it produced the crowning glory of them all. With tireless energy it blows the bubble of each individual life and then silently, relentlessly dissolves the form and absorbs the spirit into itself again.

And yet you ask, "Can chiropractic cure appendicitis or the flu?" Have you more faith in a knife or a spoonful of medicine than in the power that animates the living world?

Many of the ideas that have surfaced in the last twenty to thirty years concerning natural health have been born out of one hundred years of efforts by chiropractic to connect health care to its true foundation: the free-flowing expression of the infinite, intelligent life force. That energy, that wisdom, that radiant vitality is our birthright.

3

From Matter to Spirit: The Transformation of Peanut Butter and Jelly

A kind of super intelli-
gence exists in each
of us, infinitely
smarter and
possessed of techni-
cal know-how far
beyond our present
understanding.

—Lewis Thomas, M.D.

To understand the wisdom of the Innate Intelligence that each of us possesses, consider what happens when I eat one of my favorite comfort foods, a peanut butter and jelly sandwich. Let's say I take a bite of this sandwich. After I chew and swallow, the food drops down my esophagus (neatly avoiding my windpipe) into the stomach. Then my stomach goes to work twisting and churning, like a food processor mixing things together. It also mixes in exactly the right combination of chemicals to start to break down the food. This mixture of food and chemicals produces a glop called chyme, preparing it for the next step of processing in the small intestine.

At the base of the stomach is an opening called the pyloric valve, which squirts little bursts of the processed food into the small intestine. This is actually where we absorb most of the food's nutrients. The small intestine has its own nervous system (the enteric nervous system), which monitors the percentage of proteins, carbohydrates, and fats in the chyme, then signals the small intestine to produce chemicals in exactly the right amounts to digest each of those nutrients. The nutrients then enter the bloodstream, where they are distributed to potentially every cell in the body. You have heard that we are what we eat—well, it's true. That peanut butter and jelly sandwich has gone from my plate into my bloodstream in perhaps sixty minutes. The molecules of carbohydrate, fat, and protein have been transformed into the tissues of my body and the energy that sustains them. The question is *how* my body knows how to do that. I certainly don't do it consciously. I don't have to instruct my stomach to secrete chemicals, or direct the molecules in my intestine to seek out a particular bit of food. My conscious mind doesn't have to direct any of those functions, thank goodness, because Innate Intelligence is doing that.

▶ The Vast Wonder of Our Cells and DNA

Science tells us that there are between fifty trillion and a hundred trillion cells in the human body, and in the time it takes you to read this sentence, hundreds of trillions of chemical/electrical/biological events have occurred within the envelope of flesh you call your body. Hundreds of thousands of cells have died; hundreds of thousands more have been born. Each of your cells has been busy eating, digesting, absorbing, breathing, and eliminating—and that's just to take care of its own little bit of protoplasm. Those cells also work together to form the many biochemical factories throughout your body—such as the liver, the kidneys, and the lungs—that perform specialized chores necessary to keep the larger organism (you) alive and kicking.

Still more amazing, within each cell is an even smaller particle of matter, the nucleus, and within that is a structure called DNA.

This microscopic speck contains your entire genetic map on its twisted molecular structure. This map is in *every single cell* of your body. It is theoretically possible to reproduce your exact genetic double from any one of these cells. The more we study biology and life, the more we have to keep asking, "How does a human body know how to do what it does?" The answer, as discussed in Chapter 2, is that a human body knows what to do because of a complex relationship between our environment and its interaction with our genetic makeup, our DNA. But where does the organization arise that creates all the trillions of chemical reactions that just happened inside you and me?

I was listening to a radio program in which some of the world's top geneticists were discussing the recently deciphered map of the human genome (the structure of the genes that make up our DNA). While some of the callers commented that life was losing its mystery as a result of these scientific discoveries, the scientist said that nothing could be further from the truth. To the contrary, they were awed by this vast and complex system from which life springs. One of them even stated how he could see the handiwork of God in the current discoveries.

Much as the cellular membrane, in conjunction with signals from the cellular environment, controls and coordinates all the activity going on within each cell, the brain controls and coordinates all the activity within your body. The brain sends messages out to the organs of your body using chemical messengers called *neuropeptides.* These molecular couriers are the language used to carry on the conversation between the brain, the body, and the environment.

As I discussed in Chapter 2, one of the foundational principles of chiropractic is "Organization implies intelligence." Everything in the human body—from DNA to the almost infinite number of chemical reactions taking place at any given moment—exhibits a vast intelligence behind its astounding organization. "Thinking about the thousands of hours it would take to scientifically describe the chemical consequences of one cell's daily life," Deepak

Chopra wrote, "a neuroscientist friend of mine remarked, 'You have to conclude that nature is intelligent because it's too complicated to be called anything else.' "

Yes, from a merely mechanistic perspective, human life is nothing more than chemical reactions taking place within the body. But as I think you can tell by now, chiropractic philosophy would say life is much, much more. Chiropractic looks to and works with the intelligence that organizes and directs those chemical reactions. This master biochemist, Innate Intelligence, can transform a peanut butter and jelly sandwich into a laughing, crying, healing human being.

▶ Symptoms, Pepto-Bismol, and the Real Cause of "Dis-ease"

The philosophy of chiropractic describes Innate Intelligence as being infinite and perfect. If this vast wisdom lies within us, however, why do we have sickness and disease? This is because when Innate Intelligence is expressed as life, it is subjected to something called the *limitations of matter.* Form creates limits. When energy and intelligence are codified into the form called life, they are subject to certain universal laws—entropy, for example. Entropy is the force that breaks things down, that causes systems to lose energy and become disorganized. It is the force that ultimately brings life to the lowest state of energy possible: death.

In the human body, we see this in the natural process of wear and tear. Our cells seem to have limits built into them; they can replicate only a certain number of times before they start to decay, disorganize, and eventually disintegrate. Human beings also can accelerate the effects of entropy—through lifestyle choices, such as eating poorly, overindulging in alcohol, drinking too little water, or not exercising; through accident or trauma; or through excessive wear and tear caused by overuse of certain parts of the body. All of these things can impede the flow of Innate Intelligence through our bodies and cause us to experience what B. J. Palmer called "dis-ease." These forces also result in aging. If life and health result from Innate Intelligence expressing itself fully within a living being, then when anything interferes with the expression of Innate Intelligence, that being becomes ill at ease with itself—"dis-eased." Chiropractic philosophy would say that dis-ease always precedes disease.

A number of years ago (before I became a chiropractor) my parents went out for Thanksgiving dinner with a number of friends to a restaurant they had eaten at many times before. Upon waking the next morning they both had a fever, were sick to their stomach, and had diarrhea. My parents had been going to the same doctor for years; so they phoned him and described their symptoms. He said that they must have the flu (after all, it was "flu season") and recommended that they get some Kaopectate and Pepto-Bismol to help reduce their symptoms.

Although these drugs did reduce their discomfort somewhat, my parents' condition persisted and worsened over the next few days. When I arrived for a visit, I was alarmed at how ill they appeared. "It's okay," they assured me, "we just have a bad case of the flu."

However, the doctor's diagnosis was wrong. My parents were suffering from food poisoning. The medications they were taking actually prevented their bodies from eliminating the toxins that were coursing through their systems. As a result, my parents almost died. Luckily, the seriousness of their condition was finally discovered, and they were rushed to the hospital, where they stayed for thirteen days.

Let's look for a moment at what really happened here. First, the diagnosis was incorrect, which was partly the doctor's fault and partly my parents' fault. Giving or expecting a diagnosis over the phone is, in most instances, a bad consumer choice and a poor medical decision. Second and more important, the recommended remedy was incorrect because *it treated the symptoms and not the cause of my parents' ill health.*

It's hard to believe that over-the-counter medicines such as Pepto-Bismol can be problematic, but it's true. When a healthy body ingests tainted food, the normal, healthy response is to try to "throw off" the poison. This is how Innate Intelligence operates: If poison comes in, it tries to eliminate it as quickly and efficiently as possible. If we chemically block this process (using Kaopectate and Pepto-Bismol, for instance), the body's intelligent response has been blocked. Instead of being eliminated, the poisons continue to build up and endanger the body's health to an even greater degree.

Most of us don't like symptoms. In fact, we've been taught that most symptoms are unhealthy and should be eliminated immediately. The multibillion-dollar over-the-counter drug industry is based on this perception—and we have been educated about health in the United States primarily by pharmaceutical companies. "How do you spell relief?" "What do you do with a headache *this* big?" "Plop, plop, fizz, fizz, oh what a relief it is!" We have been taught that for every symptom there is a drug, potion, or lotion to treat it. We are left with the basic perception that our symptoms are bad, drugs are good, and health comes from a bottle. But we need to understand that symptoms are *different* from disease. For the most part, symptoms are nothing more (or less) than the body's response to a problem. In fact, in the vast majority of cases, symptoms are the means by which the body responds *intelligently* to a problem. Although not pleasant, diarrhea and vomiting are the body's healthy response to food poisoning. Fever is also a normal response to infection; the body increases its temperature to kill off bacteria and viruses. Pain is one symptom that we all dislike, yet it has many important physiological functions. Nature didn't develop our ability to feel pain because it was unnecessary. Indeed, as you'll see in Chapter 4, pain is one of the most important ways in which the body protects itself from further injury.

Having symptoms doesn't mean we are unhealthy. A healthy person can get colds or the flu and have the symptoms associated with these illnesses, but this does not mean that she is unhealthy. A healthy person can sprain an ankle and have symptoms associated with that injury. Symptoms are part of the body's natural adaptation to illness or injury. They are the means that nature has developed to heal itself.

Adaptation is one of the most important expressions of Innate Intelligence. We adapt to the changing environments that are playing on our bodies at any time. For example, when we are exposed to high temperatures, our body sweats to cool itself down. But when there is interference with Innate Intelligence, it becomes harder for the body to adapt, and symptoms and dis-ease are often the result. Germs or bacteria are a great example of this. Bacteria live on us and in us in the trillions, and yet we coexist very happily with these microscopic organisms for the most part. In fact, in the case of some intestinal flora such as acidophilus, we benefit from their presence in our bodies. But when the expression of Innate Intelligence is impeded or interfered with, then the balance between our bodies and the bacteria begins to change. All of a sudden, the germs multiply beyond our body's ability to fend them off.

The same process happens when it comes to more serious diseases. For instance, medical research has shown that damaged, potentially cancerous cells are being formed in the body all the time. Usually, however, the body's immune system fulfills its natural function by seeking out and killing these cells before they can proliferate. However, if the body's natural balance (and the flow of Innate Intelligence) has been compromised, then the immune system is less likely to do its job, and the damaged (cancerous) cells can reproduce with impunity. It is in our best interests to make sure we maintain as high a level of health as we possibly can, and that health can be best supported by making sure our bodies are functioning at peak efficiency.

▶ Health and Healing: Innate Intelligence at Work

One of the first recorded names in human history is that of Gilgamesh. He is believed to have been a ruler in the kingdom of Sumer, a region of ancient Mesopotamia. One of many myths about Gilgamesh involves his search for the most powerful herb to save the life of his sick friend, Enkidu. After many trials and adventures Gilgamesh learned about the secret herb of life and swam to the bottom of a deep lake to recover the plant. On his journey back to the city of Uruk, he stopped to rest. While he slept under a tree, a serpent appeared and ate the herb, and it was gone forever. Upon awakening, Gilgamesh wept for himself, his friend, and all of humankind.

Humankind's search for health parallels this epic myth. Every time victory seems close, somehow it slips from our hands. With each new advance and cure, a dozen new diseases seem to arise. Conventional medicine has leaped into this gap, doing what it does very well: diagnosing and treating symptoms, disease, and trauma. However, health is more than the absence of disease. You can be free of disease and still not be fully healthy. As I said earlier, disease is always preceded by dis-ease. Even the healthiest individuals are subject to forces that are wearing their bodies down. These forces may or may not be causing what we would term "disease," but they are certainly impinging upon our experience of radiant well-being and vitality. So if health is something more than just the absence of disease, how do we create it?

At the very basis of chiropractic is the understanding that true and radiant health occurs when Innate Intelligence is allowed to flow freely throughout the human body. Chiropractic is founded on a deeply held conviction that the body has the ability to heal itself. Healing is created not by taking care of symptoms, but by eliminating any blocks that impede the body's natural, free flow of energy and Innate Intelligence. Only then can the cells and tissues go about the process of healing themselves. Over time the body can be restored to a higher level of functioning—because Innate Intelligence is expressing itself as it was designed to.

▶ How Chiropractors Work with Innate Intelligence

Many people think that chiropractors are primarily back and joint doctors, but this is incorrect. Chiropractic works with the nervous system. Just as intelligent forces are holding the planets in orbit around the sun, Innate Intelligence uses the nervous system (the brain, spinal cord, and nerves) to organize the body into a complete unit. The nervous system is the body's master control system and the biological incarnation of Innate Intelligence.

Your nervous system is a true evolutionary marvel. If you look at single-celled organisms, the control of chemical activities comes from environmental signals interacting with the membrane of the cell. But as organisms evolved from single cells to more complex forms, cells took on more specialized functions, becoming tissues and organs. Simple systems for communication between these specialized cells developed, mostly involving chemicals similar to hormones. And the last system to develop, evolutionarily speaking, was the nervous system. The nervous system is an extremely fast, extremely efficient means of sending important communication throughout the entire body. Most important, it connects the body with its ultimate controller and highest concentration of information: the brain.

The main connection from the brain to the rest of the body is the spinal cord. That is the primary pathway for the flow of Innate Intelligence. If the spinal cord is healthy and whole, Innate Intelligence can express itself freely; but if there's any misalignment, impingement, or interference within that path, then the flow of Innate Intelligence is blocked. One of the most common forms of interference to the flow of Innate Intelligence comes from problems with the spinal cord and nerves—more specifically, with the joints of the bones, called vertebrae, that wrap around the spinal cord. The vertebrae protect the essential channel of nerve communication: the spinal cord. But misuse, trauma, and wear and tear can cause them to misalign or malfunction, resulting in interference with the normal functioning of the spinal cord encased within them. The term for this impingement or interference is *subluxation*. As B. J. Palmer explained it:

> *Chiropractic teaches that the life principle, or Innate Intelligence, intelligently selects and assembles chemical elements found in human anatomy; it builds organs of the body for certain purposes, and then controls and governs their function and activities by means of these mental impulses created in the brain and sent over nerves to every tissue cell in the body.*
>
> *It is obvious that impairment of the brain or nerve tissue will interfere with the normal creation, transmission and expression of mental impulses, with the result that the cells which these nerves supply will not receive or express the proper command; will not coordinate or work in harmony with the rest of the organism, and then we have the condition of dis-ease, or lack of ease.*

Chiropractors adjust the bones of the neck and back in order to remove interference with the expression of Innate Intelligence. When a vertebra becomes misaligned or joints become damaged, the nerves that run through them become "short-circuited," and we begin to get choked off from our full expression of life. By removing subluxations, the chiropractic adjustment isn't just making someone feel better; it is restoring our connection to all of life.

4

Pain and Your Amazing Nervous System: The Nature and Purpose of Pain

If your house caught on fire, would you prefer to find out when the flames come licking at your feet, or to be warned by the smell of smoke? Or better yet, to hear the piercing tone of a smoke detector long before the fire can do any serious damage? That's one of the main purposes of pain: It's nature's smoke detector, signaling us that something is wrong and to take action *now!* You put your hand on a hot stove or a fire and pain tells you to pull it back. Or you move an arm or leg past its usual range of motion, and it hurts. Pain saves us from experiencing much greater damage or injury. If you've ever gone to the dentist, gotten a couple of shots of Novocain, and then bitten your lip severely because you couldn't feel anything, you have an idea of the value of pain.

Unfortunately, sometimes a smoke detector keeps wailing long after the fire is out, and then the sound itself becomes the problem. The same thing can happen with the human body. As I will explain later, even after the stimulus that caused the pain is gone, pain may continue to course through us. At that point, the pain is no longer the signal but the dilemma we must solve as quickly as we can.

Pain is one of the great human levelers, because everyone experiences it at one time or another no matter what their age, wealth, or status. It is one of the most costly health problems in the United States, resulting in an annual outlay of close to $50 billion in direct and indirect expenses. For example, over 80 percent of the population will experience back pain at some point in their lives. Five million Americans are partially disabled by back problems, and another two million are so severely disabled that they cannot work. Lower-back pain accounts for ninety-three million lost workdays and more than $5 billion in health care costs each year. Forty million Americans have chronic, recurring headaches and spend $4 billion a year on analgesics. Arthritis affects twenty million Americans and costs more than $4 billion each year in lost income, lost productivity, and health care. And that's not counting the instances of other kinds of joint pain, TMJ (temporomandibular joint pain), cancer pain, neuralgia associated with diabetes and other illnesses, damage to the nervous system, and so-called unspecified pain (pain for which there is no apparent cause).

However, pain not only lets us know something is wrong, but it also is closely associated with many physiological responses that are part of the body's natural healing process. How we experience pain, what happens organically from the first twinge to the last vestige of discomfort, what other biological events occur when we are in pain, and why some pain vanishes quickly while other forms of pain can recur and/or linger, affecting our lives in many (mostly negative) ways—these are all elements of the story of one of the most important survival tools your body possesses.

▶ How Our Nerves Work

To understand pain, you must first understand how the cells of the nervous system transmit the pain signal. If you were to put a nerve cell underneath a microscope, you'd see little tendrils that look like roots projecting from one end of the cell body. These are called *dendrites.* At the other end of the cell you'd see a long, thin, almost cordlike structure called an *axon.* Nerve cells are linked by means of these axons and dendrites. Not through actual contact, though— the transmission of information from nerve cell to nerve cell is much more miraculous than that. As I'll explain below, nerve cell information is transmitted in the form of electrochemical impulses and neurotransmitters.

You have nerves extending through almost every single inch of your body. There are nerve cells where you'd expect them—in your toes, fingers, teeth, tongue, and so on—and a few places you wouldn't—such as the heart, liver, lungs, and intestines. Some of our nerves, like the ones that go to our skin, are designed to provide sensory information, such as temperature, pain, and pressure, to the brain. Other nerves, like the ones that go to the muscles and joints, are linked to our experience of what's called *proprioception,* or our sense of physical movement. (In truth, most of the nervous system is used not for sensation but for motor activity, and for making tissues and organs function properly.) Almost all of our nerve cells are linked in a system or network of interconnectivity that leads from every part of the body to the spinal cord and from there to the brain. Information from your nerves is processed and responded to within the spinal cord and brain (also known as the central nervous system).

The sensory experience we call pain occurs when nerve cells that are specifically designed to send sensory messages become irritated in a particular way. The message of pain travels to the spinal cord, through a kind of biological junction box, and then to the brain, where we actually interpret the message. Anyone who's in pain may find this hard to believe, but feeling pain is just a small portion of the brain's activity, comprising only 6 percent of the functioning of the entire nervous system.

Let's say you're out walking or Rollerblading, and all of a sudden you trip and skin your knee. In that moment, hundreds of biological events occur throughout your body. But what's happening with your nerves? As soon as your knee hits the concrete, the nerve cells in your skin (the organ in the body with the most widespread dispersal of nerve cells) react by sending impulses through their axons. The message travels to the very end of the axons, which then release chemicals called *neurotransmitters*. The neurotransmitters carry the information from the axon of one cell to the dendrites of the other, across gaps called *synapses*. The dendrites have receptors on their rootlike ends specifically designed to receive these neurotransmitters. Once the dendrites get the message, so to speak, they send it along to the axon at the other end of the cell, and the chain of communication continues. (Of course, all this happens almost instantaneously.)

Depending on the stimulus being provided to the nerve cell, different kinds of neurotransmitters are produced, and they stimulate specific kinds of nerve fibers. For example, the fibers excited by the pain in your skinned knee are *nociceptors*. They are what we call class C nerves, which are the smaller, more primitive chains of nerve cells. (These nerves appeared first in the evolutionary development of multicelled creatures, indicating that the ability to experience pain has been an important survival priority for most life forms from the very beginning. There are also class A or B nerves, which are thicker and communicate much faster.) Nociceptors react to several different kinds of pain or stimulation—everything from a pinprick to heat to pressure. When the nociceptors are stimulated by pain, they release a chemical known as substance P (P for pain), along with several other neurotransmitters. Substance P then carries the message of pain from nerve cell to nerve cell, through the dendrites and axons, until the message reaches the *dorsal horn,* the part of the spinal cord that's in charge of receiving data from all the sensory nerves. From the dorsal horn the injury information is relayed to the thalamus, a structure deep in the brain that's responsible for receiving sensory data and sending it on to the cortex. The arrival of substance P in the thalamus gives the brain the message, "Help! You've got pain!" so the brain can tell the body to do something about it. Then back the message goes: from the brain to the spinal cord (through a different area of the spinal cord devoted to sending messages *from* the brain *to* the body), to the nerves that branch off in the direction of the knee, all the way down to the area that was damaged when you fell. At that site, different neurotransmitters and chemicals are released that help protect the body from further injury. The knee starts to bleed and perhaps swell. The area becomes tender to the touch, and substance P continues to be emitted whenever the skin is bumped. A complex feedback loop has been established between the hurt knee and the brain, to help protect the body from having any further damage done to it.

▶ The Problems and Gifts of Pain

There is an increasing amount of research being done in the area of pain and its management, and what doctors and researchers are discovering validates the importance of pain as a biomechanism for maintaining our health. For example, substance P not only creates the pain signal that travels to the brain itself, but causes a lot of other neurotransmitters to be produced as well. It is tied directly to increased production of hormones such as adrenaline, which creates the fight-or-flight response. This is why people in pain often show increased aggression (fight) or fear and the desire to withdraw (flight). Again, this is a function of our most primitive survival instincts. When humans were still living in caves, pain was usually a very good signal that we were going to have to either fight or run like heck to protect ourselves from further injury!

The release of substance P also causes the release of other neurotransmitters that block the experience of pain. In fact, an entire class of chemical pain relievers (opiates such as morphine, heroin, and so on) are merely unsophisticated versions of the natural opioid peptides that our bodies produce. So in many cases, pain has within it its own solution—as long as the body is allowed to do what it does naturally.

A great deal of research also indicates that pain has a role to play in the healing process. These, then, can be considered some of the gifts of pain: the signal to the brain of injury or distress; the release of neurotransmitters tailor-made to alleviate our symptoms; the stimulation of the fight-or-flight survival instinct; and the acceleration of the healing process.

Does this mean you shouldn't try to relieve your pain? Not at all. Pain also has many negative effects beyond the fact that it hurts. Just as nerve cells can be found throughout the body, substance P has also been found in almost every area of the brain and body. Therefore, pain can affect the functioning of our internal organs, our bones and muscles, even our higher mental processes. That's the first problem with pain: It doesn't hurt only where the body part is injured. It also can cause decreased functioning systemwide.

The second problem with pain is caused when substance P is released over a prolonged period of time: in other words, when we have chronic pain. When nociceptors are continually stimulated, they actually become *more* sensitized to the neurotransmitter that triggers their response. It's like taking sandpaper and rubbing it on a skinned knee. Instead of there being a lessening of pain, it actually takes fewer stimuli to provoke the same response. Oversensitization to pain doesn't happen just in the injured area. The brain learns by firing a specific set of neurons (brain cells) in specific patterns over and over and over. Eventually the neurons grow more and more receptors to carry signals more efficiently, and the synaptic pathways become like well-traveled roads. The neurons themselves may also multiply, so you have more of them to handle this particular job/task/information. That's why most adults can walk much more easily than they did at two years old: Strong chains of neurons in their brains have been sending "walk" signals for years.

But here's the bad news: Your brain learns pain just as easily and quickly as it learns anything else. When you experience what's called *chronic* pain (pain over a long period of time), the neural pathways that communicate pain to your brain get larger, thicker, and more efficient. Even when the stimulus that was causing the pain is removed, you've essentially got a pain "express lane" built in your brain. Anytime even the smallest stimulus shows up, the neural pathways fire, your brain goes, "Yep, I know that—that's pain!" and passes the signal back down to the body.

One last problem: While pain is one of the body's most important signals that something is wrong, it is not always an accurate signal. *The amount of pain you experience is not necessarily proportional to the severity of an injury.* Some life-threatening conditions—high blood pressure or diabetes, for example—rarely have pain as one of their symptoms. Many severe injuries, where people are shot or stabbed, can cause very little physical pain, even if there's been significant physical damage. In many cases of chronic pain there are no readily detectable injuries that could cause the problem; in this case, pain is not a symptom, but the problem itself.

This means that you can't use pain, or the lack of it, to gauge your overall level of well-being. That's like driving your car for a hundred thousand miles and never looking under the hood, changing the oil, or checking the tires, but thinking that everything is okay just because none of the warning lights are on. Health is not merely the absence of pain, although being pain-free is a component of feeling healthy. True health is so much more than that. And it's our responsibility to take care of ourselves long before we get that pain light on our body's dashboard.

▶ Why Chiropractic Succeeds Where "Treatment" of Pain Fails

If pain is communicated primarily through the nervous system, and chiropractic's main focus is to restore the nervous system to optimal functioning, it should be clear why chiropractic care can be a very effective way to treat pain even though pain relief is not chiropractic's main focus. Yes, most people initially seek chiropractic care for treatment of pain. Yes, many chiropractors advertise treatment of pain, and indeed, many pain problems are resolved by chiropractic care. But fundamentally chiropractic is not a pain-treating modality. What chiropractors do is restore proper motion or position to the bones of the back and neck. This removes interference to nerves, restores proper joint function, and decreases muscle spasm along with a whole host of other benefits. One of the side effects of these benefits is the reduction or elimination of pain. In essence, chiropractic treats pain without trying to.

When you go to conventional medical doctors for treatment of pain, what choices will they offer you? Drugs or surgery for the most part, with the occasional advice to rest the affected area in the case of sprains or strains. But what are most drugs designed to do? To stop pain receptors from doing their job by intersecting chemically somewhere in the cycle of pain creation that I described above. There are opiates such as morphine and heroin, salicylates such as aspirin and other nonsteroidal anti-inflammatory drugs (NSAIDs), as well as a range of medications designed to mimic the body's natural pain suppressors. But the drug companies have yet to come up with a medication that acts exactly the same way as the body's natural pain-suppressing chemicals. The drugs we have are gross imitations of what the body provides, and unfortunately these gross imitations often come with serious side effects, especially when used over a long period of time. For instance, every year in the United States 76,000 people are hospitalized and 16,500 people die directly as a result of taking NSAIDs, which have been linked to internal bleeding and digestive problems. Aspirin has long been known to affect the stomach negatively, and morphine, heroin, and the other opiates bring with them a strong risk of addiction.

Conventional medicine falters even more when it comes to the treatment of chronic or long-lasting pain. Most of chronic pain is associated either with terminal illness, such as cancer pain, or more often with neuromusculoskeletal problems, including back pain, neck pain, the pain of carpal tunnel syndrome, or the joint pain of arthritis. Treating chronic pain with drugs or surgery is all too frequently ineffective, or worse—it can cause more injury than the original complaint. Only a few years ago, bed rest and anti-inflammatory medication were the standard medical prescriptions for back pain. But now research has demonstrated that this approach causes *more* disability.

The key to true recovery is *restoration of function.* The best way to alleviate back pain is to get the patient moving, which helps to restore normal functioning to the bones, muscles, and connective tissue. That's basically the approach chiropractic has used for decades; however, the functioning that chiropractic wants to restore is much more subtle than most conventional medical doctors would recognize. When pain in the neuromusculoskeletal system is addressed through chiropractic, which focuses on restoring function rather than treating pain, the pain erases or disappears with no drugs or surgery required.

In chiropractic we also say, "Pain is the last thing to show up, and the first thing to go." When there are problems in the spine and nervous system, pain is frequently the last symptom to show up, especially if the damage is caused not by trauma (like a car accident) but by improper functioning of a particular joint or vertebra. For example, if you have a back problem related to some kind of misalignment or slight shift in the spine, the first thing you notice may not be pain but a slight restriction in your normal movement. You feel a little stiff, or you can't touch your toes anymore, or your neck doesn't move from side to side quite so easily. The normal, optimal functioning of your spine or neck has been compromised, but you may or may not experience any pain until the condition gets a lot worse.

If you have a repeated abnormal functioning—using your shoulder to hold the phone by your ear, for example, or sitting at the computer with your wrists held at an uncomfortable angle, or holding your head in an abnormal position for long periods of time because the computer screen is off to the right, down too low, or up too high—over time the joint malfunction causes continued microdamage to the joint. This can go on for a long time before pain occurs, and by then you've got permanent damage to tissue.

In another circumstance, perhaps you do have a fall or an accident that causes pain, and you take care of it with analgesics, ice, and massage. Once the pain goes away, you stop treatment. But the accident has also caused a loss of functioning in the affected area. By treating only the pain, you are not restoring normal function.

Pain also is usually the first symptom to disappear when someone begins chiropractic treatment; and that's unfortunate. Why unfortunate? Pain often disappears long before the underlying condition is healed and normal functioning is restored to the body. That's one of the reasons most chiropractors prescribe a course of treatment that goes on even after patients have no more pain, because chiropractic is focused on correcting the malfunctioning that created the pain in the first place. The chiropractor wants to restore you to health and optimal function, not just take away your pain.

Think of optimal functioning and extreme pain as being at opposite ends of a continuum, like this:

0% Function	30% Function	40% Function	100% Function
Extreme pain	Noticeable pain	No pain	Optimal functioning

Depending on your particular condition or damage, you may have only 40 percent function and still be without pain. Pain may not occur until your level of function drops below 30 percent, and that's when you go to see your chiropractor. The chiropractor helps you get to 45 percent functioning, and you no longer have any pain. But are you functioning at an optimal level? No. What's more important, how small is your margin of error at 45 percent? You can lose only 15 percent of functioning before you experience pain again. On the other hand, if you continue care and get to 85 or

90 or 100 percent functioning, you can handle a lot more physiological stress without pain because your margin is so much greater.

Chiropractic's approach to treating pain without treating pain is much more sane and sensible than the conventional medical approach. Yes, chiropractic is absolutely interested in helping patients with their pain, but rather than treating the symptom called pain, they treat the cause by restoring optimal functioning. Remember that skinned knee we talked about? If you were just to treat the pain, you'd take a couple of aspirin or get a painkiller shot and that'd be it. But could you do only that and restore your knee's ability to function? No—you have to clean the knee, put some antiseptic on it, make sure there's no foreign matter lodged in the abraded area, and then put a bandage on it. As the scab formed, you'd have to keep moving the knee to make sure the joint wouldn't freeze up or the scar tissue wouldn't be so tight that you couldn't bend the knee. Are any of those actions focused on relieving pain? Not really, although they may help. They're more about restoration of function, getting the knee back to where it was. Chiropractic restores function, and pain relief is the logical consequence. And wouldn't you like *both* pain relief and optimal functioning, without having to resort to drugs or surgery?

5

The Secret of Chiropractic: Releasing Your Body's Self-Healing Power

Perhaps you have seen chiropractors at county fairs or local stores, performing spinal screenings. They may be using everything from postural analysis machines to more sophisticated computerized muscle-testing devices. My associates and I have done such screenings for many years in Washington State. Our purpose is to educate the public about the importance of spinal health and chiropractic care, and we have been able to help many people as a result.

Marcia was one such person. While shopping in a local superstore, she saw one of our screening booths where my associate, Janet, was working. As Marcia and her husband, Jim, passed the booth, Jim said, "That's just another chiropractor trying to peddle her services. You don't want to stop there." But later on, when they walked by the booth again, Marcia decided to get a screening just for fun.

While performing the necessary measurements, Janet asked Marcia if she had any specific complaints. "No more than the usual aches and pains of someone in their fifties," Marcia replied. "But I was wondering if chiropractic could help my high blood pressure." This was a condition she had suffered with most of her adult life. Traditional Western medicines had been of no help; either she had a terrible reaction to the drugs, or they simply didn't work for her. After the test, Janet explained that while chiropractic care was not a treatment for high blood pressure, Marcia's screening indicated some spinal imbalances. She recommended that Marcia come in to our Health First offices for a more comprehensive exam.

I am happy to say that Marcia did indeed become one of my patients. After Marcia received a few adjustments to the upper neck, her blood pressure went through some wild swings for a few weeks, then settled at a level that was the lowest she could remember. This was a remarkable experience for Marcia, to say the least, but the benefit didn't stop there. My wife and I occasionally meet Jim and Marcia for breakfast, and the conversation usually veers in the direction of chiropractic. At one of our breakfasts, Marcia admitted there was more to her chiropractic story. "I never thought much about how stiff I was every morning, how hard it was to reach my feet as I tried to put on my socks and shoes," she told us. "It wasn't until I woke up one day and realized that those problems were gone that I understood that chiropractic had benefited me on more levels than I could even know." Although chiropractic helped Marcia with her blood pressure as well as other health problems, her blood pressure did not reduce to the level that her medical doctor wanted, even with diet and other lifestyle changes. Eventually she did find a medicine that reduced her blood pressure to acceptable levels without side effects. This is a good example of how modern medicine can be used in conjunction with alternative approaches.

In numerous studies, chiropractic has proven to be one of the most effective treatments for back pain, neck pain, many types of headaches, and other musculoskeletal ailments. Additional studies show that, while not a panacea, chiropractic care can be an effective treatment for a variety of health problems ranging from chronic tonsillitis to high blood pressure and many other conditions (see Appendix I). How is this possible? Because chiropractic removes subluxations—blocks in the spine to the normal flow of information, energy, and intelligence from the brain to the rest of the body—it can help resolve a number of conditions that you might not associate with the spine or nerves. Once you understand the workings of the spine and nervous system, the effect of subluxations on overall health becomes all too clear. And to understand the spine and nervous system, you need to see how these miraculous structures develop from our earliest beginnings in the womb.

▶ The Body's "Information Superhighway": The Spine and Spinal Cord

We begin life as a mass of cells that are the result of the union of an ovum and sperm. When an embryo starts to form inside a woman's body, all of its cells are undifferentiated—that is, identical to one another. However, as these cells continue to divide, the embryo develops three layers: top, middle, and bottom. There is a slight differentiation between each layer, but still nothing yet that resembles an organ or a specific tissue. And then, around the nineteenth day after conception, directed by Innate Intelligence, this disk of cells folds in on itself and creates the very first recognizable organ: the neural tube, or *notochord,* which eventually will become the baby's spinal cord.

Around the third or fourth week, as the embryo continues to differentiate, a brain stem and a little nub of a brain appear at one end of the notochord. Then the nervous system tissue begins to sprout: Nerves grow out of the spinal cord, and cells begin to differentiate and form around the nerve branches, like buds on a tree. These buds will become arms, legs, bones, muscles, internal organs, and many other structures of the body. At the same time the primordial formation of the gut occurs, buds appear that will turn into the lungs, and the vascular system also begins to develop.

All of this is happening as part of the genetic expression of the embryo in its development. But for much of the developing embryo, it is the nerves and nervous system that direct the growth of tissues and organs. Sometimes growth is initiated by the nervous system; in other instances the nervous system comes in later on and regulates development of tissues after they've originally formed. Sometimes nerves grow for a while and then disappear! While a fetus is in the womb, many nerves and structures appear, perform a function, then melt back into the extracellular tissue.

Scientists say, "We don't know why this happens," but I believe the answer is obvious: The nerves and nervous system are the primary conduit of Innate Intelligence, which is directing the development of this fetus. Certain nerves may grow for a while to help with the development of whatever organ/tissue is needed, and when that organ/tissue reaches a certain level, the nerve disappears. The nervous system is the master control center; without a nervous system, the fetus would be a mass of cells communicating very poorly with each other.

Just as Innate Intelligence has created and developed specialized functions in the cells, tissues, and organs, it has created a system—the nervous system—that specializes in information and energy. Nerves lead from almost every single part of the body to the spinal cord, and from there to the body's seat of intelligence—the brain. Much the way the bones of the skull protect the brain, the spinal cord is protected by the bones of the spine, called vertebrae.

The spine is one of the most complex organs in the body, consisting of nearly a hundred intricate joints connected by a vast array of ligaments, tendons, cartilage, and six layers of intertwining muscles, all surrounding and protecting over a trillion nerve pathways that connect the brain to the rest of the body. This complex network of tissue is the structural foundation for the vital mind-body connection. The spine is a unique structure within the human skeleton, in that it is designed to have enormous mobility, flexibility, and strength. It not only provides the strong protection of bone, muscle, and tendon for the fragile spinal cord, but it also serves as the anchor and entry point for nerves from almost every single part of the body.

For organizational purposes, most medical texts and doctors (including chiropractors) divide the spine into five parts. The cervical area, or neck, consists of seven small bones extending from the base of the skull to the top of the shoulders. The twelve bones of the thoracic area, the largest section of the spine, extend from the shoulders through the midback. The lumbar area, or lower back (a spot where many back pain complaints occur), contains five large vertebrae. The sacral area below it consists of five fused bones. Finally, the sacrum is connected to the three fused bones of the tailbone, or coccyx.

Each section of the spine has various sets of nerves running to it and away from it, and misalignments in each area can create different symptoms and conditions. Some chiropractors believe that misalignments in the cervical area have a greater impact because they impinge on communication from the brain to the rest of the body. Others ascribe to the viewpoint that problems in the sacroiliac or lumbar area are most important because they form the structural foundation of the spine. Regardless of these different technical approaches, virtually all chiropractors share the conviction that it is important for the bones of the spine to maintain proper alignment and function. This ensures the uninterrupted flow of Innate Intelligence and energy throughout the body.

▶ When Communication Is Blocked

The brain is not just the seat of mental intelligence; it is also the seat of our body's intelligence. How do we know this? Simple—if the nerve connection between brain and body is compromised, the area to which the nerves go is affected. That's why injuries to the spinal cord are so serious: They can affect all the organs, limbs, muscles, and bones that usually send and receive information through the injured area. The arms and legs of paraplegics and quadriplegics are typically not what has been injured; their problems are usually due to a spinal cord injury. The limbs are not receiving instruction anymore from the brain and the central nervous system. Therefore, they no longer function as they should.

Luckily, most of us will never experience a severe injury to the spinal cord. But lesser injuries happen all the time. Babies' necks get twisted during the birthing process. Children fall off tricycles or bicycles, or out of tree houses. Adults have auto accidents, or sports injuries, or simply get up from a chair the wrong way. And it's not just injury to the bones of the spine that causes misalignment. Damage to the soft connective tissues surrounding the bones of the spine can be equally problematic. This is because once these tissues are damaged, the vertebrae can lose their correct alignment or proper mechanical function. *Any* impingement of the bones of the spine and the surrounding connective tissue can interfere with the nerves. When this happens, it not only can cause pain and loss of function in the back, but also can affect other areas and organs. These impingements, or subluxations, choke off the ability of Innate Intelligence to control and coordinate body functions through the nervous system.

One of the easiest ways to visualize this process is by thinking of a safety pin. The safety pin not only represents one of the most elegant and functional designs you'll see in an everyday object, but also serves as a very clear depiction of how the brain and body communicate. The clasp end of the pin represents the brain, and the other end where the metal loops around is the target organ. You have nerves that lead from the brain to the target organ (called *afferent* nerves), and nerves leading from the target organ to the brain (*efferent* nerves). As long as the safety pin is closed, communication can flow from the brain (clasp) to the target organ (loops) and back again. But if the pin is opened, the connection is broken, and communication no longer flows efficiently. That's what a subluxation does: It causes a short circuit to the brain-body nerve connection, and communication is impaired as a result.

Conversely, when the spinal bone is put back into alignment, communication can flow once again. The body's natural self-healing mechanisms are activated. The nerves, organs, and affected areas begin to return to their proper level of functioning, and we experience renewed health and vitality. The chiropractic adjustment closes that safety pin, thereby allowing the body to do what it does naturally—heal itself.

▶ Subluxations: Subtle Yet Serious and Prevalent Blocks

In conventional medicine, *subluxation* refers to a misalignment of any bone, but in chiropractic, a subluxation is anything within the area of the spine that breaks the cycle of nerve communication between the brain and the body. It's like a short circuit in the body's nervous system. It used to be that chiropractors, like conventional medical doctors, believed that misalignment of vertebrae put direct pressure on the nerves and the spinal cord, and this pressure caused the symptoms associated with subluxation—pain, loss of range of motion, and many other effects on nerves and organs throughout the body. However, with advances in molecular research and the ability to study the biochemical processes of the body, we now understand much more about the mechanism of subluxation. We also understand why so many different types of chiropractic treatments can be helpful regardless of the particular method used.

A subluxation is usually caused by a trauma to the spine—either an incident such as a fall or accident, or a repeated abnormal biomechanical movement over time. When the trauma occurs, there may or may not be a visible shift in the alignment of the vertebrae, but there is almost always a change or reduction of the range of motion in that particular vertebra. Think of it as beads on a string. They move around on the string and slide freely up and down. If for some reason, however, you get a kink in the string, the beads can no longer move freely. They bump into one another;

they get stuck in a particular position. They don't have the same *range of motion* as they did before the kink.

That's what can happen with the bones of your spine. Vertebrae don't have fixed positions; instead, they have a *range* of positions that they are designed to be able to take comfortably. (Otherwise, you wouldn't be able to bend, turn your head, or lean side to side.) If one of your vertebrae gets out of alignment due to trauma or repetitive abnormal motion, the kink usually affects the normal movement capacity of the bone. Then, like Marcia, you might experience stiffness, a reduced ability to turn your head to one side or the other, soreness in your back, and so on. You may or may not experience pain, but there will definitely be some kind of effect on the health of the body.

But the effect of a subluxation doesn't end there. When a subluxation occurs, the trauma or injury not only can cause misalignment of bone, but it also creates damage to the soft tissue surrounding the vertebra—ligaments, tendons, cartilage, and muscles. These are called the *connective tissues,* and most vertebrae have six different "joints" or groups of connective tissue connecting them to the bones above and below them. Damage to connective tissue usually takes the form of microscopic rips and tears in the localized area and produces a range of uncomfortable symptoms including muscle spasm, swelling, and inflammation. The symptoms can be either *acute* (happening for a short time and then disappearing after treatment) or *chronic* (recurring over a longer period of time). If the damage is not corrected, the connective tissue between the vertebrae can wear away, allowing the soft cushion between the vertebrae to bulge outward (a herniated or ruptured disk). When this occurs, the vertebrae press upon the spinal nerves and create tremendous pain. In truth, it is the damage to the soft tissue and not to the vertebrae themselves that most often interferes with the proper functioning of the nerves and the spinal cord.

When the connective tissue swells, it also has an effect on the biomechanics of the bone it surrounds. Let's use a misaligned neck vertebra as an example. Say you were in a car accident and experienced a minor amount of whiplash. The third or fourth bone in your neck is now slightly out of alignment, and you're experiencing discomfort, swelling, and tenderness in the area. The swelling of the connective tissue prevents you from moving the misaligned bone correctly, even if you could. The combination of misalignment and localized tissue damage generates what we call *abnormal biomechanics* in the joint—which simply means you're moving your neck in a reduced range of motion, probably in ways the joint was not designed to function. And here's the real problem: Moving your neck in this abnormal way causes more damage, more microtears, more buildup of scar tissue that locks in the incorrect position and motion. Or perhaps the pain and swelling cause you to stop moving the joint altogether, producing what's called *disuse atrophy* in the connective tissues as well as the muscles surrounding the joint.

▶ The Mechanism of Injury

Now, what happens in the body when an injury occurs? The body's defenses rush in and quickly start to replace any damaged tissue. But as with any other kind of rush job, the body is less concerned with quality than it is with getting the job done. So instead of replacing the damaged tissue with exactly the same kind of cells, it lays down what we know as scar tissue.

The same process happens in the connective tissue surrounding the vertebrae. When injury occurs, the body's defenses rush in and start laying down cells to replace the damaged ones. (This is called *infusion of scar tissue.*) However, these new cells are larger, grosser, and much less well organized than the ones they are replacing. Instead of being laid down in nice, neat rows, the scar tissue cells fill in the holes any way they can. Especially if there is a decrease in the range of motion of the joint, the scar tissue is a chaotic, jumbled mass of cells. And just like a scab on your knee, the scar tissue in your connective tissue isn't as flexible as the cells it's replacing. That's why a subluxation can create a lasting decrease in the range of motion of a particular joint—it's as if the effects of the misalignment are being cemented in with the formation of scar tissue in the connective joints.

Eventually, the scar tissue in your joints is replaced by finer and finer grades of cells (just as the scab on your knee is replaced by pink skin, then by almost normal skin). It can take anywhere from six to eighteen months for a soft tissue injury to remodel itself fully, but the replacement tissue is never going to be identical to the tissue that was damaged in the first place. There will always be a slight decrease in quality. However, there are things you can do to help the healing process and actually assist your body in laying down organized tissue instead of disorganized scar tissue. Chiropractic care is one, and we'll be talking about other ways to help your body heal in Part II of this book.

▶ Subluxations, Short Circuits, and Inflammatory Soup

What we have reviewed above relates primarily to local tissue injury around the subluxated vertebra. How, then, does this local problem cause widespread nervous system interference? First of all, subluxations can affect the flow of cerebrospinal fluid throughout the central nervous system. Cerebrospinal fluid is a liquid that flows around the different sections of the brain and through the spinal canal, providing protection and nutrition for the spinal cord and nerves. Any impingement or obstruction of the flow of cerebrospinal fluid can prevent proper communication from one end of the spinal cord to the other and interfere with the function of any or all of the nerves that attach to the cord. It's like trying to make a cell phone call in an area where there's a weak signal. You might be able to make every third or fourth word heard, but you'll have a hard time getting your entire message across, or hearing the response from the person you called.

The second systemwide problem caused by subluxation has to

do with what are called *feedback loops.* Current research shows that the trauma associated with misalignment sets in motion the production of chemicals that cause swelling and inflammation in the local tissue (as noted above). This is part of the body's normal response to tissue injury. These chemicals bathe the local nerves, causing a profusion of nerve receptors to fire, thus overloading nerve pathways. The overloaded nerves send a barrage of signals straight to the dorsal horn of the spinal cord. These messages are then sent to the brain. Once the signal of distress reaches the brain, the brain sends signals back down the spinal cord to the affected area. A feedback loop has now been created between the injured joint, the spinal cord, and the brain. The brain is telling the body to handle the problem in the affected area, and so new chemicals rush in to help.

Here is where one of the problems arises: Unless you correct the cause of the injury, the affected area will continue to send out distress signals in the form of floods of neurotransmitters. The brain will try to help but won't be able to correct the subluxation. Because of muscle spasm, torn or damaged tissue, infusion of scar tissue, and the nerve interference itself, the self-healing capacity of the body will be overwhelmed. Instead of getting better, the injury will either stay the same or get worse. Until we assist the body in breaking this cycle of distress, we are doomed to either a subtle or obvious loss of function and health.

But the real problem doesn't just distress the injured area. The inflammatory soup also is affecting the nerves going to the spinal cord and brain. The nerves in the affected area are flooding the central nervous system with neurotransmitters that are spilling over into other nerve pathways in the spinal cord and brain. This in turn can affect information being transmitted throughout the body. The effects can show up in your arms, legs, hands, stomach, lungs—almost every area and organ in the body. The self-healing feedback loop has been broken; the hormones and neurotransmitters the body uses to take care of inflammation and all its other problems are not doing their job. Instead, a feedback loop of detrimental chemical and biological reactions is taking place, making things worse rather than better. Until the health of the nervous system is restored and proper motion returned to the vertebra, the body is in crisis, unable to handle the normal wear and tear of everyday life. It can't fight off infection; it has trouble digesting or assimilating food; perhaps it becomes more sensitive to toxins in the air or water. If the nervous system is not functioning properly, the health of the body is seriously compromised.

Unfortunately, subluxations occur frequently, and may or may not have obvious causes or symptoms. Think back over your own history of bumps, bruises, and less obvious injuries. That fall you took out of a tree house when you were nine? Maybe you've had headaches since that time and never associated the two occurrences. The sore neck you have when you leave work? The hours you spend with the phone cradled between your ear and shoulder may be pulling your neck out of alignment. The old football injury? Competitive sports are one of the biggest causes of subluxations. Whether caused by childhood injury or yesterday's misstep off the curb, the problem of subluxation is pervasive. Studies have found that there is some sort of spinal imbalance in 80 percent of twenty-year-olds and 95 percent of forty-five-year-olds. That means *subluxation is the single most widespread health problem on the planet today.* There is no other single condition that affects more human beings. Sadly, only 10 percent of the U.S. population is currently receiving regular chiropractic care, which means that somewhere between 75 and 85 percent of people are walking around on the streets today with their brains partially choked off from their bodies.

If left untreated, subluxations can cause the muscles, bones, and nerves to degenerate. This degeneration appears in many different forms: osteoarthritis, thinning of disks, formation of bone spurs, muscle weakness, and nerve interference that can cause numbness and lack of function. The effects of subluxation can range anywhere from causing no symptoms at all to causing death. Unless you are getting regular chiropractic care, you may find yourself continuing on a path of diminishing vitality, greater discomfort, less mobility, and mounting health complaints. These are not simply symptoms of aging, by the way (as we are taught by most conventional medicine). They may very possibly be the effect of old subluxations. Handle the subluxations, and you might well find your health greatly improved.

Remember Marcia from the beginning of this chapter? You wouldn't think that subluxations in her spine could have any relation to her high blood pressure. But blood pressure is regulated by the *autonomic nervous system*. These nerves (which are divided into two categories, the sympathetic and parasympathetic) are responsible for the body's involuntary functions, such as heart rate, blood flow, contraction of the muscles that move food through the intestines, glandular activity, and so on. If the function of the autonomic nervous system is being impaired by subluxation, then correcting the subluxation would allow the nerves to resume their task of regulating involuntary functions like blood pressure. In Marcia's case, her high blood pressure was reduced following a course of chiropractic care.

Let me give you another example of how subluxations can impede functioning in different parts of the body. A few years ago Andrea walked into my office complaining of severe headaches two to three times a week and sciatic pain running down her left leg. I diagnosed a severe subluxation at the C1 level (the C1 is the vertebra at the very top of the neck, where the spine joins the skull). Andrea told me later that she didn't really believe that adjusting her neck would help her leg pain. But she decided to give chiropractic a try for six weeks, on the off chance it would help her headaches. Sure enough, within six weeks Andrea's headaches had become far less frequent. More important, however, her leg pain had disappeared entirely. Why? Andrea had been suffering from a tilted pelvis, which was pinching her sciatic nerve. When the C1 was adjusted, the pelvic tilt resolved and the pressure on the sciatic nerve was relieved.

In my practice I see patients like Andrea and Marcia all the time—people who come in for conditions such as back pain, whiplash, headaches, and so on, and who are amazed to find that their other health problems are eased or eliminated with regular chiropractic care. But when you remember that chiropractic treats nerves rather than bones, and that nerves connect with almost every other organ and system, then it makes complete sense that correcting subluxations can help restore health and vitality throughout the body.

▶ How a Chiropractic Adjustment Works

There are many ways you can intervene in the cycle of inflammation and injury that accompanies a subluxation. A conventional medical doctor might prescribe anti-inflammatory medication, which stops the production of the neurotransmitters creating pain and swelling. This intervention might give the body's self-healing systems a chance to get in there and do the repair work necessary to reduce inflammation naturally. But unfortunately, repair work takes time, and with anti-inflammatories you're treating not the *cause* of the injury but a *symptom.*

Let me give you a concrete example of what I mean. Say you take a rubber band and wrap it around your finger several times so that it's uncomfortably tight. What would happen if you left the rubber band around the finger? The circulation would be cut off, and eventually the tissue of the finger would die. Now let's say that you couldn't see the rubber band. (Of course we *can* see the rubber band, but in reality many of our health problems result from interference to normal function that we can't see.) Long before the finger died you would know something was wrong with it. Why? Because it would hurt!

Now, perhaps you go to a conventional medical doctor, and he can't see the rubber band either. (It's not his fault; he hasn't been trained to look for rubber bands.) You tell the doctor, "My finger hurts." The doctor replies, "You have pain? No problem. I can fix pain." And he gives you a shot of local anesthetic.

A week later you return to the doctor and say, "That pain reliever you gave me was really good stuff, but there's still something wrong." And he answers, "Okay, we'll look a little closer." So he examines the finger and says, "Hmmm, the color of that finger doesn't look too good. I don't think you're getting proper blood flow. We'll use a drug called a vasodilator that will open up the veins and arteries."

Do you know the difference between a medicine and a poison? In many cases, the only difference is dosage. Although the vasodilator may work temporarily, if you take too much of it, it can kill you. And remember, the rubber band is still around your finger.

So back you go for another visit. You tell the doctor, "You know, that medicine you gave me helped a little bit, but this finger still isn't right." He says, "Okay, it looks like we have a major blockage here, so we'll have to do bypass surgery. We'll cut a vein and an artery on each side of the blockage and sew them together to bypass the blockage." Will that solve the problem? No—the rubber band is still there.

How do you solve the problem with your finger? *Take the rubber band off!* Treat the cause of the problem, not the symptoms. That's what chiropractic does: It is specifically designed to treat the cause—the subluxation itself.

Chiropractic philosophy says that in a large percentage of cases of illness, the body doesn't need anything added to or taken away from it. What's needed is to remove interference with normal physiological function, and then the body can heal itself. A chiropractic adjustment, even though it's a force from the outside, is designed to remove interference with normal function. When this happens, the connective tissue returns to normal. The adjustment moves the bone through a range of motion that has many physiological benefits. This motion helps the joint to flush out the inflammatory soup and restores the release of neurotransmitters to proper levels. The nervous system is then allowed to do its job of transmitting messages smoothly between brain and body. And the vast majority of patients find their health and well-being improved.

Although many patients feel relief following an adjustment, the effects may not be immediate. It takes time for the body to restore itself to optimal functioning. But by addressing the subluxation rather than the symptoms, the chiropractic adjustment allows the body to activate its self-healing mechanisms. With this interference removed, healing happens at its normal, natural, most effective pace.

Typically most people think the adjustment moves the bone from an abnormal position back into place. This is not precisely what happens. Remember, a vertebra is not fixed; it is a bone-joint complex that has a normal range of motion. With a subluxation, the bone can't move properly. Either it's locked outside its normal range, or it has been patterned into an abnormal way of moving. The adjustment is designed to unlock the joint from its locked position or abnormal way of moving. It does this by gently pushing the joint beyond the lock, to the limit of its passive range of motion. At times when the joint is pushed beyond the lock you'll hear a slight popping sound, as if you were cracking your knuckles. This is nothing to worry about; it simply indicates a release within the joint. The sound is often followed by a sensation of relaxation. If you've ever done stretching exercises, either yoga or part of a warm-up routine, you know how it feels to stretch a muscle to its farthest point and then go a little bit farther. That's similar to what the adjustment does. It helps the joint remember its normal range of motion.

To see what I mean, try this experiment. Take one of your hands and point your index finger straight up at the ceiling. Now, try to arch your finger back as far as you can. It probably doesn't go far— a couple of degrees. This is called the active range of motion. Now, use your other hand to push gently back on that finger. How much more can you arch it back? You can probably take it another 20 to 30 degrees without any pain. This extra movement is referred to as the passive range of motion. In virtually all joints the passive range of motion is greater than the active range. If you push into the passive range of motion, it doesn't hurt anything, because it's within the realm in which the joint is designed to function.

When somebody has a subluxation or a fixated joint, it's typically fixated in less than its active range of motion. In other words, you can't even move it as far as you normally would by using your own muscles. Limiting movement in this way is one of the body's means of protecting itself from pain. However, a limited range of motion causes the formation of disorganized scar tissue and results in ongoing abnormal motion in the affected area. To heal the cause rather than the symptom, you need to restore normal range of motion to the joint. The chiropractic adjustment takes that joint and moves it back into its active range of motion and then to the full extent of its passive range of motion.

Here's the good news: If the normal range of motion is restored quickly following an injury, it will affect the way new tissue forms in the injured area. Instead of a chaotic mass of scar tissue, the new cells are laid down in lines associated with the stress of normal motion. Reintroducing motion helps the joint heal better and stretches the new cells as they are forming. The new tissue forms in a way that accommodates proper functioning of the joint.

The other symptom commonly associated with a fixated joint is muscle spasm. When a joint becomes locked, the muscles around it lock up, too, holding the joint even more firmly in place. The thrust and motion of the chiropractic adjustment interrupts the muscle spasm, breaking the feedback loop and allowing the muscle to relax. Once the loop is broken, the muscle can then return to its normal state, allowing the joint to move more freely.

Finally, and most important, the adjustment also helps to flush out the inflammatory soup and restore normal communication between nerves and the spinal cord. It's almost like pushing the reset button on your neural computer, because it normalizes the neurological function in the area. As the spine and the nervous system heal, Innate Intelligence once again flows clearly, quickly, and cleanly throughout the body, as it was meant to. The body naturally begins to let go of stored pain and disease. And you can start to experience the level of health and vitality you were always supposed to have.

Now that you understand the philosophy and basic principles upon which chiropractic care is based, I hope you have made the decision to explore chiropractic as one of your own health care choices. But as in other health care fields, there are specialties and subspecialties in chiropractic. In the next section you'll learn about choosing the chiropractor and the kind of treatment that's right for you. Chapter 6 will give you a broad overview of the different kinds of chiropractic care available, and how to find a practitioner whose focus will suit your needs. The rest of the section will show you how to work with your chiropractor in attaining the highest level of health and well-being.

PART II

The Practice

6

Choosing the Chiropractor
Who's Right for You

Imagine you want to eat some fruit, but you have none in the house. For most of us, that means a trip to the supermarket. But that's only the first in a chain of decisions that you need to make. Do you want fresh, frozen, or canned? If fresh, what kind of fruit? Oranges, apples, pears, peaches, melons, and grapes are all on display in the produce section. If your taste is for apples, what variety do you prefer? Some people like apples that are sweet; others like a bit of tartness; still others base their choice on crispness. And those who want to bake apple pie have an entirely different set of criteria for the perfect apple.

Choosing your health care provider involves a similar but much more serious chain of decisions. You begin by making the biggest choice: to go to a conventional medical doctor or to explore a route that focuses more on creation of health than on diagnosis and treatment of disease. Your decision may also be based on the type of problem you are having. If you opt for the health-promoting side of the marketplace, your next option has to do with the different kinds of care provided by what's called alternative medicine. You might wish to visit an acupuncturist, naturopath, colon hydrotherapist, homeopath, nutritional counselor, and so on. If you're reading this book, I believe you have chosen or are considering chiropractic care as part of your health care program.

Even within chiropractic care, there are choices to be made. While most chiropractors correct subluxation and restore normal biomechanical function, within the field of chiropractic care there are approximately forty to fifty different major techniques that are used. The level of force and the area of the spine focused on can vary from technique to technique. Some chiropractors specialize in fields such as sports chiropractic, accident recovery, or cranial manipulation. The different techniques are based on a wide variety of scientific discoveries and theoretical assumptions about joint mechanics and muscle and nervous system function, and each technique has value in certain circumstances. A chiropractor's style of practice also may reflect his or her philosophical inclination.

For purposes of choosing a chiropractor, however, you only need to understand that all chiropractic care falls into three general categories. In this chapter you'll learn about each one, and how to ask questions of any practitioner you want to consider as a health care provider. I've also included a sample interview you can use when talking to practitioners.

Choosing a chiropractor isn't complicated. The most important things you can do as a consumer are to (1) know the kind of treatment and/or care you want, (2) seek out practitioners who will offer that care, and (3) ask questions to determine if this particular doctor fits your needs both personally and professionally. Since many chiropractors consider patient education a vital part of their job, they are usually quite delighted to give you all the information you need to make an informed choice. After all, chiropractic care is a partnership in creating health, and for a partnership to work both partners must participate.

▶ Straight, Mixing, and Allopathic Chiropractic

The terms *straight* and *mixing* have been used to describe two traditional schools of chiropractic thought. *Allopathic* chiropractic is used to describe a more recent direction some practitioners have taken. Straight or "subluxation-based" chiropractic is most closely related to the original premises of B. J. Palmer. It regards subluxations of the spine as one of the primary causes of ill health in the body, and its practitioners focus very closely on using the chiropractic adjustment to eliminate subluxations and restore the flow of Innate Intelligence. Subluxation-based chiropractors offer adjustments as their specialty. They may recommend that their patients receive massage or physical therapy to support the effects of adjustments, but they will not usually expand their practice beyond these areas. The straight school of chiropractic believes that the body has the ability to heal itself with the least amount of intervention. "All we do is adjust the bone, remove the nerve interference, and then allow the body to heal," they say. "We simply adjust the subluxation and then let the body take care of the rest. The more precise the adjustment, the greater the benefit." Subluxation-based chiropractors consider that they have a focused scope of practice, and their expertise is in adjusting the spine. Although they believe the health benefits of this focused approach are widespread, they do not offer themselves as a replacement for traditional medical care.

Mixing chiropractic, on the other hand, refers to those practitioners who choose to perform additional services for their patients beyond adjustments. A more modern and descriptive term for these chiropractors would be "broad scope" practitioners. A broad scope chiropractor asserts that while treatment of subluxation *may* still form the primary treatment of a patient, there are other modalities that can support the correction of the subluxation and the healing process. Broad scope chiropractors often draw upon a wide range of alternative and conventional medical techniques as part of their practice. Some of them offer medical diagnosis, iridology, homeopathy, naturopathy, massage, nutritional counseling, and sometimes even emotional and behavioral support. If you choose a broad scope chiropractor, you may receive another kind of treatment in addition to, and sometimes instead of, an adjustment. Correction of subluxation is only one modality among a number of other therapies. But all broad scope chiropractic treatments still aim to restore the health of the body naturally. This approach offers a one-stop option for the patient and is often viewed by the practitioner as a replacement for traditional medical care.

Most chiropractors fall into either the subluxation-based or broad scope schools of thought. The third category, allopathic chiropractic, is focused primarily on treatment of symptoms. (*Allopathic* is a term used to describe conventional Western medicine.) Many allopathic chiropractors believe that their job is not to correct subluxation but to treat back pain. They may even question the existence of subluxations. Like conventional medical doctors, allopathic chiropractors are focused more on relieving symptoms through the use of whatever means are necessary, as opposed to correcting underlying causes. They usually treat a patient for five to six sessions, and if he or she isn't getting better, they refer the patient to an orthopedic physician, usually for surgery or drug therapy.

The kind of chiropractor you choose depends on what you want from your chiropractic care. If you want someone who specializes in adjustments and only adjustments, and who probably has an exceptional degree of precision and experience in doing them, then a subluxation-based chiropractor is your best choice. If you like the idea of bringing in a wider range of treatment options from the alternative medicine field, or if you're already familiar and comfortable with another kind of alternative care, such as homeopathy, you may wish to find a broad scope chiropractor who has knowledge in that area. If you want only relief from pain and feel most comfortable with the kind of symptom-based care offered by conventional medicine, then an allopathic chiropractor might suit your needs. It all depends on the kind of care you wish to receive and what you are most comfortable receiving.

When choosing your chiropractor, there are a few basic questions you can ask that will help you determine whether this practitioner is right for your needs. In the next few pages I'll discuss what you need to know to select the best doctor for you.

▶ Does the Doctor Focus on a Particular Part of the Spine?

As you learned in Chapter 5, the vertebrae of the spine can be divided into five different sections. Over the years, different schools of chiropractic technique have focused on treating specific areas of the spine. One group may focus on the hips, sacrum, or lower back, based on the view that the spine is built from the bottom up. Others say that we are built neurologically from the brain down, therefore the upper neck is the most important area. Then there's a general school that doesn't differentiate between sections when it comes to focusing their treatment.

Chiropractors who specialize in upper neck work mainly adjust the top two bones of the neck. They believe that misalignment in this area has a much greater effect than subluxations located elsewhere in the spine. Their reasoning is based on anatomy. The upper neck is the area that's closest to the base of the skull and the brain stem. Subluxations in this area can affect communication throughout the central nervous system at the highest point possible in the spine, thereby blocking signals to the entire body. Those in this school of thought say that if the upper neck is properly adjusted, the rest of the spine will heal itself. Their objective is to get patients better with the fewest adjustments needed to create better long-term stability, and with less dependence on continuing chiropractic care. Although upper cervical chiropractors are only a small percentage of practitioners, their work is often considered some of the most precise and potent.

Chiropractors who focus on the lumbar or sacral area take the opposite view—literally. They believe that subluxations in the lower spine affect the structural stability of the entire spine, just as a weak foundation might threaten the structural integrity of an entire home. There are also neurological implications created by subluxations in the lower spine. At the lower end of the spinal cord is a structure called the *cauda equina,* a bundle of nerve roots that emerge from the spinal cord and spread out like a horse's tail (thus the Latin name of the structure) and travel into the lower abdomen, reproductive organs, and legs. There is some indication that subluxations in this area can affect the flow of cerebrospinal fluid throughout the central nervous system. Thus, instead of interfering from the top down, the interference is from the bottom up.

If you go to a chiropractor who doesn't give special weight to any one area of the spine, he or she will do adjustments throughout the entire spine. The chiropractic approach you choose depends on your needs and your comfort with the doctor's philosophy. While some patients like the idea of getting as few adjustments as possible and thus may choose a chiropractor who specializes in one area, others feel like they want to get it all done. In reality, most chiropractors employ a variety of approaches to suit both the clinical needs and personal preferences of their patients. The difference between one chiropractor and the next is more a matter of where their starting point is (the top or the bottom), and whether they tend to be more aggressive (a lot of adjusting) versus more conservative (as little adjusting as possible).

▶ How Much Force Is Used?

Chiropractors differ not only in the areas of the spine they focus on, but also in how much force is used while adjusting. Of the many chiropractic techniques, most are primarily different ways to provide a specific kind of adjustment to the spine. Since many techniques are similar, as a consumer, you don't really need to know which technique your chiropractor is using. But you might want to know the level of force involved.

Some chiropractors use very low force in their adjustments. They make use of what are called *trigger points*. Trigger points are specific locations on the spine that are connected energetically with different organs and limbs. Because trigger points are very sensitive, applying even small amounts of force at those locations will create significant changes in the organs and limbs that are connected with them. (Based on ancient Chinese medicine's knowledge of energy flow, trigger points also are used in acupuncture, acupressure, and reflexology.) Other chiropractors make use of pressure probes or wands, again to apply a light force in very specific areas. Many chiropractors who focus on cervical and upper cervical work use primarily low-force techniques. Because the bones in the neck are relatively small compared to other vertebrae, a very slight adjustment can have a significant effect. Other low-force techniques you may hear chiropractors refer to include Toftness, DNFT (directional non-force technique), and Logan technique, which applies low-force adjustments to the bottom of the spine.

Most chiropractic adjustments fall into the medium-force category, with a few moving into what would be considered high force (although high-force adjustments are rare). Medium-force adjustments utilize the principle of long or short levers. Long-lever adjustments usually involve pressure applied to a "long lever" such as a leg, arm, hip, or shoulder. The body is torqued, or twisted, to bring the affected joint to the point in its range of motion where it's locking up. Then a quick thrust is applied to move the joint past that point, thereby unlocking it and restoring its normal range of motion. If you imagine somebody lying on the table on his or her side and the chiropractor pulling one leg up over the other one and then giving the upper leg a quick thrust, that's a medium- to high-force adjustment. Sometimes these adjustments are accompanied by a slight popping sound as the joint is unlocked. This is nothing to worry about—it's similar to cracking your knuckles or feeling a pop in your jaw while chewing gum.

Short-lever techniques take a more subtle approach. Rather than torquing or twisting the body, the patient is kept in a neutral position, usually lying facedown on the table. Instead of applying pressure to the leg, arm, or shoulder, the chiropractor puts his or her hands right on the affected vertebra and pushes on it in a very specific direction. Often this type of chiropractic utilizes a piece of equipment called a *drop table*. Drop tables are intricately constructed so that different sections of the body can be positioned at a particular level. When the chiropractic thrust is applied, that section of the table drops by a certain amount in response. The drop is only a small amount, less than an inch. Using a drop table actually makes the adjustment less forceful and more precise, as the table absorbs most of the energy of the adjustment.

In some cases, chiropractors will find it necessary to use high-force adjustments to free a joint or bone that is locked in such a way that medium force will not release it. The principle of long-lever adjusting is used, but the chiropractor applies more energy to the thrust. High-force adjustments are rare, however, since most chiropractors prefer to use the least amount of force necessary to release the joint and eliminate the subluxation.

It's useful to know the level of force your chiropractor uses for the adjustments. If you go to a low-force chiropractor expecting a more forceful adjustment, you probably will be disappointed. On the other hand, if you are sensitive to pressure or pain, or if you are worried about having an adjustment for any reason, a low-force chiropractor may seem gentler and more suited to your needs. The good news is that most chiropractic techniques work regardless of their level of force, the equipment used, even the area of the spine to be treated. Which one you choose is simply based on your own individual taste.

▶ Interviewing Your Chiropractor: A Few Simple Questions

There is a wide variety of thought and approach within the realm of chiropractic care. I believe this is one of the strengths of the profession, because it allows for ongoing, vigorous, and thought-provoking discussion within the ranks. It gives you, the consumer, greater choice. But it also gives you more responsibility. As with all your health care providers, you have to take charge, do your research, and ask questions.

If you have been referred to a chiropractor by a friend (as many people are), you might begin by talking with your friend about his or her experience of chiropractic care. But remember that your friend is probably not an expert and may have no idea about the technique, focus, or philosophical bent of the chiropractor. So no matter how glowing a recommendation your friend may give chiropractic, do your own research.

Luckily, unlike far too many conventional doctors who rarely seem to have time to talk with their patients, most chiropractors regard patient education as one of the most important parts of their job. In my experience, chiropractors are usually happy to answer your questions. Many allow a no-charge consultation for new patients, which offers you a face-to-face encounter with the doctor while giving you an idea about how the office is run. If you are investigating a number of chiropractors and want to make a general assessment before meeting a doctor face-to-face, a telephone interview may also be useful. But whether you're on the phone or in the chiropractor's office, feel free to use the Chiropractic Interview questions in this chapter. They should take no more than about five minutes to answer, and will help you select a chiropractor who closely matches your needs and expectations.

I'd be cautious about a health care professional who is "too busy" to answer your questions. Of course, any practitioner may not be able to talk at the moment you call, but he or she should be available to return your call or to schedule a consultation with you. It is only through communication and education that doctors empower patients to take responsibility for their own well-being. And a doctor who respects your desire for information and wishes to create a relationship of communication and caring is the only kind of health care partner you want to have on your journey through life.

Chiropractor Interview: Suggested Questions

A. *General information*

1. Does your work focus on adjustment of the spine or do you offer a variety of modalities, like nutritional counseling, homeopathy, massage, and so on?

2. If other modalities are used, what are they, and why do you use them?

3. Is the care at your office focused on:
    a. Short-term pain or symptom relief?
    b. Medium-term rehabilitative care?
    c. Lifetime health maintenance care?

4. How do you work with other health care practitioners? Do you refer to conventional medical doctors if necessary? Do you have other alternative practitioners you will refer me to if I ask?

B. *Technique-related information*

1. Do you offer specific adjustments or more general mobilizing manipulations?

2. Does the primary approach/technique you use have a specific name?

3. Can you give me a brief description of your adjusting technique?

4. Is your primary adjusting technique low-force, medium-force, or high-force?

C. *Symptom-related questions*

1. The symptom(s) I have is (are) _____. What is your experience in helping people with this problem?

2. Can you give me an estimate regarding the percentage of patients who have had this problem and have gotten better under your care?

3. How long can I expect it to be before I begin to feel better?

4. If my problem does not respond to chiropractic care in the expected time frame, what would be the next step I should take? Will you refer me to another practitioner and work with them?

▶ Making Chiropractic Part of Your Total Health Care Plan

Choosing a good chiropractor is an important part of your health care—but only a part. You should be open to using both alternative and conventional medicine to support your overall well-being and vitality. As a chiropractor, my job is to focus on correction of subluxation; it's not my objective to provide all the care someone needs. I prefer that my patients have a good team of doctors working for them, including a conventional medical doctor, a dentist, perhaps a nutritionist or a naturopath, and other specialists as needed. The key is to find doctors who are willing to support a team approach to your health. More and more allopathic medical doctors are becoming open to the benefits of alternative medicine, so when choosing your primary-care physician, make sure to ask, "Do you work with health care practitioners like chiropractors?" (In fact, with a few small changes, you could use the questions in the Chiropractic Interview to evaluate any health care provider— conventional, alternative, or in between.) If you find your current allopathic doctor discourages the use of alternative means of health care, you may wish to find one who is more in tune with your own ideas about health.

In this era of skyrocketing health care costs, chiropractic care is still relatively inexpensive. Although it is important to know what your current health insurance will cover, in some cases it may be necessary to go outside of your insurance to get the care you need and desire. Insurance was originally designed to avoid catastrophic financial losses, not to pay for every health care cost that arises. Throughout the United States and Canada, most insurance coverage includes chiropractic care. (The more innovative plans will even allow you to use a chiropractor as your primary-care physician.) Of course, some plans are better than others, and many will only pay for acute care, not care designed to restore full function and maintain health. If you wish to make chiropractic a part of your regular health care regimen, you may need to do a little research and consider that at least some of your care will have to be paid out of pocket. Most chiropractors have payment plans and financial arrangements to suit family health care needs. But whether or not you have health insurance that will cover all of your chiropractic needs, the increased health and vitality you will gain from regular chiropractic care will be well worth the expense.

The bottom line is, *be informed.* How you take care of your health is your choice, so make sure that you become an informed and active consumer of conventional and alternative medicine alike.

7

What to Expect from Chiropractic Treatment

Conventional medicine is a passive experience for most patients. When you go to your medical doctor, usually you first describe your symptoms. Some tests may be run, and then you may be given a drug. Your entire role in the process has been to point the doctor in a specific direction to guide his or her diagnosis, take whatever's prescribed for you, and pay handsomely for the privilege.

Chiropractic, on the other hand, involves teamwork, with you and your doctor as equal players. Chiropractors usually request that you take an active role in every part of your health care relationship with them. Often there are classes to attend, videos to watch, literature to read, and perhaps exercises to do. Much of what is asked of patients is based on chiropractic philosophy, which states that

100 percent health comes from 100 percent expression of Innate Intelligence. Since health comes from the expression of Innate Intelligence flowing freely through the body, it is not something that can be imposed from the outside. Therefore, the patient is responsible for his or her own experience of health.

Chiropractic care has been in the forefront of the movement toward natural health and patient responsibility for over a century. Chiropractic recognizes patients as equal partners in their health decisions. The chiropractor is not there to dictate but to educate, guide, and inform patients about achieving optimal health. But patients must do their part, through lifestyle choices and maintaining some kind of regular health care regimen.

In this chapter we'll walk you through what you can expect from your first few visits to the chiropractor you've chosen. We'll talk a little about X rays, why many chiropractors feel they're essential in providing you with the best level of care, and how X rays today are safer than ever. We'll go through the treatment process and begin the discussion of what I call the "chiropractic lifestyle"—making health choices to create and maintain optimal vitality and well-being through the years.

▶ What to Expect During Your First Visit

Once you've chosen your chiropractor, you'll make an appointment for an initial consultation and exam. In our offices, we presuppose that any new patients will have questions about chiropractic, and we have created a series of events to educate patients as soon as they walk in the door. But most chiropractors will have at least three goals for your first visit: (1) gathering information about you, (2) giving you basic information about chiropractic, and (3) creating what the doctor hopes will be a long-term health partnership between patient and practitioner.

Most people are very pleasantly surprised when they walk into chiropractic offices, because they are far more friendly and welcoming than what they may have experienced with other health care providers. There is usually a waiting area and reception desk where someone will greet you and confirm your appointment. If it's your first visit, the receptionist will also give you paperwork to fill out. In our offices, the paperwork comes with a cover sheet explaining what will happen during your first visit.

In addition to the standard contact and billing information, most chiropractic patients are asked to complete a personal health history. This may include questions regarding their primary complaint, general health, lifestyle, and family health history. As you understand by now, chiropractic care potentially can help a wide range of health problems that on that surface may not be associated with back or neck pain. So if you experience any kind of chronic condition—from asthma to digestive problems, high blood pressure, or problems with your eyes—make sure to include the information in your health history or mention it to your chiropractor.

After you've completed all the paperwork and returned to the receptionist, you may see the doctor right away, or you may sit with a chiropractic assistant who is trained in the basic diagnostic elements of chiropractic. The assistant will review your health history with you, then present the main points to the doctor prior to your seeing him or her. The assistant might also talk with you briefly about what to expect from the doctor and give you some general patient education information. In our offices, we request that all new patients watch a ten-minute video on their first visit, to give them a brief introduction to the principles of chiropractic philosophy. Other doctors give patients some reading material or a pamphlet to take home following their consultation.

Next, you'll probably meet the doctor, who will give you a series of physiological tests. These may include general health evaluations, like blood pressure, height, and weight, and will undoubtedly feature tests to evaluate the condition of your spine. Some of the tests you may receive include:

1. *Postural analysis.* The doctor may observe you standing to see if you're standing straight or slouching, favoring one leg over the other, holding one shoulder higher, or tilting

your head to one side. This is called a *visual postural analysis.* Some doctors use a frame designed to measure variations in posture from one side of the body to another; others have fairly high-tech equipment that uses computer imaging to assess posture.

2. *Neurologic testing.* This may include reflex evaluation, where the doctor taps on your knee or elbow with a small hammer, for example, or pinwheel testing, where a small metal pinwheel device is run across different areas of the body to determine sensitivity or numbness.

3. *Orthopedic testing.* Here the doctor may gently twist, turn, and bend different joints to see if there is any discomfort. For example, he or she may ask you to bend your head to one side and then will press on it gently, to see if extending the movement is uncomfortable. Some chiropractors who adjust the extremities as well as the spine may take you through a series of orthopedic checks for a particular area of complaint, such as the elbow or knee.

4. *Range of motion tests.* The doctor will ask you to bend and turn your neck and back, to determine the current range of motion of the joints. Sometimes the evaluation is done visually; sometimes a protractor (like the ones you used in geometry class, only bigger) will be used to measure the angle of motion available to a particular portion of the neck and back.

5. *Thermographic analysis.* Many chiropractors use some sort of heat-reading or thermographic instrument to measure skin temperature and then compare readings on each side of the body. This reading is actually a neurological test: Skin temperature is determined primarily by blood flow to the skin, and blood flow is regulated by the sympathetic nervous system. Elevated skin temperature on one side of the body can indicate excess nerve activity in that area. (Hippocrates was one of the first to use skin temperature as a

diagnostic tool. Physicians at his school used to put wet clay on a patient's back, and then they would watch which areas would dry first. The areas that generated more heat indicated a potential problem. If you've ever experienced inflammation in part of your body, you're familiar with the sensation of heat that emanates from the area.) Chiropractors have been using heat-reading instruments for about sixty years, so there are different types of thermography your doctor might employ. If you don't get a thermographic reading, however, don't be concerned, as not every doctor uses this measurement.

6. *Motion palpation.* This is a very specific range of motion test, where the doctor puts his or her hand along the patient's spine and rocks back and forth in different ranges of motion. By feeling the spine, the doctor can detect abnormal joint mechanics of different vertebrae.

In addition to testing, the doctor will undoubtedly ask a number of questions about your general health and any chronic or acute complaints, as well as observing your level of comfort or discomfort while standing, sitting, and moving. All these tests are designed to allow the chiropractor to measure your current state against a perceived norm, and to come to the most complete and accurate diagnosis possible. The testing you will receive depends both on the doctor and your particular condition. If you've just been in a fairly significant auto accident, for example, the chiropractor will run different tests than if you're walking in with a chronic problem. But most chiropractors will use some sort of combination of orthopedic and neurological testing to evaluate your current physical condition.

▶ The X-Ray Question

The other test you may receive as part of your chiropractic evaluation is an X ray of the spine. Nowadays a number of people are concerned about the overuse of X rays in all medical professions, and I know of no chiropractor who takes X rays lightly. At the same time, the value of X rays as a diagnostic tool for chiropractic is immense. Because so many chiropractors use X rays in their practices, as a profession, we have done our best to keep up with all the technological advances that have made X rays much lower in dose and safer in the past several years.

Why are people concerned about unnecessary X rays? Because each X ray is a dose of radiation, and they have heard that the exposure is cumulative. Therefore, the more X rays they receive, they think, the more likely they are to have problems with radiation sickness. But the kind of radiation in an X ray is different from the kind that makes you radioactive. The radiation that makes you radioactive is referred to as *nuclear* radiation, and it comes from the nucleus of atoms of elements such as uranium and plutonium. X rays, on the other hand, are *ionizing* radiation: The electromagnetic force used in X rays comes from the electron shell of the atom, not the nucleus. Therefore, the radiation of an X ray is more closely related to light and radio waves than it is to uranium. In fact, you could sit in front of an X-ray machine all day long and be bombarded constantly with X rays and never become radioactive.

There are reasons to avoid unnecessary X rays, however, that have nothing to do with radioactivity. The moment an X ray passes through the body, its energy can knock electrons out of the atoms it comes into contact with, causing damage to soft tissues on the molecular level. This damage to tissue eventually could cause some forms of cancer.

There are three things that need to be taken into account when considering the damage that X rays can cause. First, the tissues that are the most likely to be damaged by X ray are those that reproduce quickly, including the skin and the reproductive organs. (This is why pregnant women are cautioned against having X rays, because the fetus is a mass of quickly reproducing cells and thus is vulnerable to the radiation.) Other types of cells, such as bones, muscles, and nerves, do *not* reproduce quickly and are not as susceptible to damage by X rays. Therefore, as long as precautions are taken to protect the reproductive organs, most X rays taken by your chiropractor can be considered fairly safe.

Second, with the current advances in X-ray technology, the amount of radiation needed to get an accurate picture of your spine is very low. One kind of technology, intensifying screens, is a great example of these advances. It works something like this. If you compare an X ray to sunlight, you can think of an X ray as a very bright light that's capable of shining through your soft tissues but not through the denser bones inside. The bones would then cast a shadow, just as your body does when you stand outdoors in bright sunlight. If you put a light-sensitive piece of film on the other side of the body from the source of the X ray, the shadow of the bones will be cast on the film and captured there. It used to be that the radiation of the X ray would cause the film to be exposed and the image imprinted. But now the X ray falls on something called an intensifying screen, which has been impregnated with rare earth chemicals that glow when exposed to minute amounts of X-ray radiation. When the X rays hit the screen, the chemicals glow brightly enough to expose the film behind them. The film used is also much better, requiring much less exposure time to record an image. Thus, the amount of radiation used in one X ray today is about 90 percent *less* than it was even ten years ago. You would probably have to have hundreds of X rays taken within a sixty-day period to be in the danger zone. In fact, you receive more electro-magnetic radiation on a flight from Seattle to Los Angeles than you do in a year's worth of X rays at your chiropractor's office!

Third, it's important to remember that any kind of X-ray testing is subject to very strict state regulations, to which every medical professional—conventional doctors, dentists, chiropractors, and so on—must adhere. These regulations are designed to protect the health and safety of both consumers and the people who give the X rays. No one wants patients to be subjected to unnecessary X rays, and as a conscientious health care consumer, you should always be willing to speak up and ask about any procedure or test.

At the same time, you must be willing to weigh the benefits and the risks of any test as objectively as possible.

Some chiropractors don't include X rays as part of their diagnostic support testing because they feel such tests are not needed for the kind of adjusting they offer. The only reason these doctors might take X rays is to rule out cancer or other conditions that might contraindicate adjustments or require referral for other care. Many low-force doctors, for example, don't use X rays; the amount of force they use in their adjustments is such that they aren't worried about contraindications that might appear on an X ray. There also are some chiropractors who question whether subluxations are even visible on an X ray. Their reasoning is that a subluxation is not a static condition but one that appears when the joint is in motion, and therefore no static picture (like an X ray) can clearly depict it. Another section of the profession says, "No, you actually can see structural aberrations or subluxations on an X ray, and you can use the film to indicate the direction in which you should push the bone."

It's up to you which choice you prefer: X ray or no X ray. However, I wouldn't adjust without X rays. First of all, the work I do (primarily in the upper neck area) is very precise, and the best way for me to evaluate the exact location of a subluxation is with an X ray. Second, current research on chiropractic adjustments seems to indicate that any adjustment force should be in line with the way the bones of the spine are articulated, or linked one to the other. Because everyone is made just a little bit differently, the only way to determine a patient's unique structural makeup is with an X ray. Third, I prefer to err on the side of safety and precision. Especially when it comes to the cervical vertebrae (which are much smaller) or the lumbar area (where you run the risk of disk problems), I insist on taking X rays before beginning treatment.

That being said, there are some areas of the spine that I *would* feel comfortable adjusting without seeing an X ray, simply because the vertebrae in these areas are more stable. The midback and hips, for example, are pretty easy to evaluate for subluxation without X rays, and are fairly easy to adjust. In addition, there are some consumers whose problems can be resolved without a lot of precision. Here's what I say in my patient education classes: "For about 20 percent of the people who come into my office, I could tell them to bend over and grab their ankles, then hit them on the butt with a shovel and they'll be cured. In those cases, the body simply is waiting for a force to come and fix it, and all I'm doing is supplying the force. Another 20 percent require a slightly more specific application of force. I could feel around and then give them a general, high-force, long-lever adjustment and resolve their condition quickly. Another 20 to 30 percent will need more diagnosis. I'll need to do physical testing and X rays so I can give them a more precise and specific thrust on a specific bone in a specific direction in order to fix the problem. The last 20 percent of patients are the difficult cases. With them, the more precise the adjustment, the higher the rate of success. But when someone walks into my office, I don't know if they're part of the 20 percent where I could hit them in the butt with the shovel or the 20 percent where I'll need to be extremely precise. So I have to assume that everyone is in the difficult 20 percent."

B. J. Palmer once said, "Chiropractic is specific or it is nothing at all." Any tests your chiropractor gives you, including X rays, are designed to allow him or her to give you the most precise adjustments possible. Precision means safer adjustments, more specific outcomes, and a larger number of people who will profit from chiropractic care.

Back to your first visit: At this point, the chiropractor may request X rays of your entire spine, or perhaps only one portion. This is not just for the purposes of diagnosis and being able to provide precise adjustments; it also will help establish the outcome of your treatment. Remember, as I said in Chapter 1, chiropractic care focuses not on the relief of symptoms but on the *restoration of function*. When you go to a conventional medical doctor, the outcome of treatment is usually pretty obvious: The symptoms— pain, fever, nausea, and so on—will go away. But with chiropractic (and good science), it's important for the doctor to have clearly defined, objective, measurable outcomes. And one of the best ways to establish outcomes is for the patient (and the doctor) to see his or her current condition on an X ray.

▶ A Typical Patient

Typically the first visit is devoted to diagnosis and assessment of the patient's current condition. Unless someone is in extreme pain, many chiropractors won't adjust the patient until the second visit. Much of the second visit focuses on what's called "report of findings and outcome assessment": explaining to the patient what's going on with him or her, and the course of care the chiropractor recommends.

Let's take the example of a typical patient, John. John was in a minor car accident. His neck hurt for a few days and then the pain went away. (This is typical in low-impact rear-end collisions occurring at speeds between 5 and 20 mph.) But over the next few weeks John started to experience chronic neck pain, and his vision was a little blurry. One of his golfing buddies suggested that John come to see me: "Dr. Lenarz really helped me when I hurt my back last year," the golf buddy said. John decided to make an appointment at my clinic.

On his first visit John received a thorough examination and workup, including X rays. I interviewed John, went over his medical questionnaire, and performed some of the tests described earlier in this chapter. Then I asked John to return three days later, when I would give him a report of findings, outcome assessment, and adjustment. John left my office with some reading material covering all the basics of chiropractic care.

Three days later John returned to my clinic.

"Well, John, looks like you're having some fairly serious problems with your neck," I told him. I put John's X ray on the light box and pointed to the image. "A healthy neck should have a gentle, forward-sloping curve to it. As you can see, yours is pretty straight. That's probably due to the whiplash, or it could be a result of abnormal tension of torquing from sports or work. Were you ever in the military?"

"Yes," John said.

"It's also called 'military neck,'" I replied, "because men and women in the military are asked to stand and hold their heads in such a way that forces the normal curve out of the neck."

I put an X ray of John's lower back on the light box. "You also have a few subluxations in the lower back that we should take care of as well. They may or may not be due to the auto accident, but they are definitely impinging on your spine. I've put all my findings and recommendations in your report."

I handed John a folder, on the front of which was his name and the words "Report of Findings and Outcome Assessment." The report included a list of all the areas of the spine that were being impinged upon and a diagram of the entire spine and neck with each affected vertebra indicated. On a separate page all of John's symptoms were listed, along with my summation of what he wanted from his chiropractic care. I reviewed the goals with John. "You told me you want to eliminate the pain and gain mobility in your neck, and you want to get rid of some of the stiffness you say you feel after golf sometimes. To achieve those goals, I'll adjust your neck over a period of time to restore its normal curvature and range of motion. We'll also work specifically on the lower back to handle any abnormal torquing caused by golf. That should eliminate your current symptoms, but more important, you should feel much healthier and more mobile overall."

John agreed with the outcomes and then asked, "How long do you think it will take?"

I replied, "That depends on how well you respond to treatment, and that varies from patient to patient. I recommend that you come in three times a week for the first two weeks. The third week we can cut back to two visits and continue with those for about a month. After that you can come in once a week until the three-month mark, at which point I'll take another set of X rays to evaluate your progress. Eventually you'll go on a maintenance program, where you come in once every two or three months just to take care of normal wear and tear."

"I thought I was just coming in to treat a sore neck," John commented. "But I guess there's a lot more involved."

"Chiropractic care isn't just for handling emergencies; it's designed to keep you healthy throughout the year," I said. "It's just like taking care of your teeth. If you'd had a tooth knocked out in the auto accident, you'd go to your dentist, and he or she would put it back, or replace it with a crown or implant. But that wouldn't mean you could stop going in for a cleaning and checkup every six months if you want your teeth to stay healthy. To keep your back and neck healthy you need regular chiropractic care. So are you ready for your first adjustment?"

John agreed, and I took him into my adjusting room. Some chiropractors' offices resemble conventional medical offices, with a series of little rooms suitable for treating one patient at a time. Others more closely resemble a physical therapy room, with open adjusting bays where several patients can receive treatment in the same space. I have a room with open adjusting bays, and separate rooms where patients can rest after the adjustments. I walked John over to one of the adjusting benches. "I don't want you to think I'm going to sneak up behind you and adjust you," I said. John laughed, and I continued, "So let me explain what's going to happen. In a moment I'm going to have you lie down on your side on the bench, and then we'll do the adjustment." Because I use drop tables when I adjust, I showed John exactly how the table would work. I raised the headpiece of the table and demonstrated how John would rest his head on the headpiece. Then I showed him the small amount of thrust I would apply to his neck by putting my index finger on his shoulder and pressing down. "That's all the energy I'll be using," I said. "Pretty gentle, right? The adjustment happens very quickly and it might be a little startling, but it won't hurt." I applied the same amount of pressure to the headpiece, and John could see how the headpiece would drop by about a half an inch when I did so. "The headpiece actually absorbs most of the energy of the adjustment," I told John. "That way you'll receive the gentlest adjustment possible."

John seemed reassured and climbed willingly on the table. The adjustment was over in a few seconds, and he was astounded. "That's it?" he said.

"In 90 to 95 percent of cases adjustments are a gentle experience, and even the ones that are relatively high-force are not painful," I said. "Now I want you to lie down for about twenty minutes and rest." (While I do this in my practice, it is not typical.) "Before you leave, make sure you set up your appointments for the rest of your initial program."

"The adjustment was a piece of cake, Dr. Lenarz," John said. "But I've still got a little neck pain. Should I be worried?"

"Usually after an adjustment about 40 to 45 percent of people feel better, about 50 percent don't feel much difference right away, and about 5 percent actually get a little extra stiff and sore," I answered. "During their first week of care most people usually have about three days where they feel better than they have in some time, and they'll also have about three days when they feel a little extra stiff and sore. That's because once we start adjusting, the rest of the body begins to adapt to the new or proper position of the bone. And as the rest of the body begins to shift and change, some things can get a little bit stiff and sore. But give your body time to establish a normal, healthy balance and I think you'll be pleased with the results."

John followed his treatment plan religiously, and his symptoms improved steadily as he continued to get adjusted. He still had a few rough days, but, as I told him, that was to be expected. He wasn't just getting rid of the effects of the accident; he was eliminating problems he had had for ten or more years. John's chiropractic wasn't a quick fix but a long-term course of care. Within two months, however, John reported his golf swing had improved because he no longer had back and neck pain. Within three months he was able to move to maintenance care, where he got adjusted once a month. (Because John plays golf, he needed monthly rather than quarterly adjustments.) And now he's telling his own golf buddies about the benefits of chiropractic.

I have described John's case in detail so you will have an idea of a typical course of care. Naturally, your own treatment will depend on your spinal condition and symptoms. The course of care recommended by your chiropractor most likely will include a series of adjustments, or it may be "Come in three times next week and then we'll see." During each visit the doctor may adjust you once or treat several areas of your neck and back. The doctor may also suggest other treatments to support your overall health. Depending on your specific condition, your doctor may recommend physical therapy, massage, Rolfing, nutritional counseling, or other modalities. Again, the length of treatment and the elements included will be based on your particular physical condition, and what the chiropractor believes is needed to restore your body to optimal functioning.

▶ Cycles of Healing

Life is full of cycles. Everything alive comes into being, grows, and eventually dies: That's the cycle of life itself. On the microscopic, molecular, and chemical levels, virtually all biological processes are cycles, from the ATP cycle (the process that releases energy stored in our muscles) to the Krebs cycle (how cells take in oxygen and use it to create energy) and the reflex mechanism in our nerves. The human body is composed of cycles within cycles, within the larger cycle of birth, growth, and death. Many of these cycles interact with one another. For instance, the Krebs cycle requires vitamin C and a number of different chemicals that are produced by other processes within the body. Most of these cycles occur in a matter of milliseconds. The science of biochemistry is based on an understanding that these chemical cycles are taking place all the time.

Injury and healing are combinations of many different cycles. While the initial injury can happen very quickly (like breaking a leg or skinning a knee), there is a cascade of biochemical responses following the incident that affect not just the injured area but virtually every system within the human body. To truly heal after an injury requires that all systems be restored to their normal levels of functioning.

There's an old truism that you can tear down a building a lot faster than you can put one up. This is equally true of the healing process. Restoring damaged tissue takes more time than it took for the effects of the injury to be felt. And just like putting up a building, certain things have to happen in a specific order for your body to withstand the forces of nature. Suppose you decided you wanted to put the roof on your building before you had dug the basement, or thought you could hang Sheetrock before you put together the wooden frame that supports the walls! Your house wouldn't stand very long, would it? In the same way, the human body has to do very specific things in a very specific order to heal completely. If it doesn't, you can end up with even more trouble than was caused by the original injury.

The processes that regulate healing are controlled by Innate Intelligence, and cycles of healing are very much a part of chiropractic philosophy. Do you remember the safety pin cycle we discussed in Chapter 5? The clasp end represents the brain, the wires represent the nerves, and the end where the wires loop around represents the organ or part of the body the brain is communicating with. As long as the body is healthy, information can flow smoothly from brain to body and back again in a cycle. But if something interferes with communication—if the safety pin is opened for any reason—the communication cycle is broken.

A subluxation is any interference to this communication caused by problems in the vertebrae or the soft tissues that support them. However, as we also learned in Chapters 4 and 5, the effect of a subluxation extends beyond a simple misalignment of bone. There is almost always injury or damage to the soft tissue around the vertebra. Subluxations also produce negative effects on the areas of the body or organs at the other end of the "safety pin" nerve connection. For example, a subluxation of a vertebra that interferes with a nerve leading to your foot might produce numbness, tingling, or pain in that foot. If left unattended for long enough, there could even be some damage to the nerve or foot itself. Because the nervous system controls tissue function, if you interfere with nerves going to a target tissue, the cells of the target tissue *and* the extracellular matrix the cells live in begin to become unhealthy. As a result, the cells stop repairing themselves and replicating properly. Those cells will continue to replicate themselves in an unhealthy manner, creating unhealthy and diseased tissue.

When the subluxation is corrected and proper function is restored to the nervous system, the nerves and the target tissue begin to heal because you are bringing those cells and tissue back to their normal function. However, it might take a while for full function to be restored. Indeed, even in some cases where full nerve communication eventually returns, the damage caused in the interim may be too severe to be healed fully. That's one of the reasons why regular chiropractic care is so important: We want to catch and treat subluxations as early as possible to prevent the likelihood of permanent tissue damage.

The good news is, chiropractic adjustments allow the body to do what it does naturally: heal itself from the inside out. By correcting subluxations, chiropractic adjustments start the process of healing by restoring the spine to its normal position, thus allowing all the associated soft tissue, nerves, and target organs to begin healing as well. Adjustments launch the body's healing cycle, and continuing adjustments support the body in its journey back to health.

Healing a skinned knee happens pretty quickly and easily, but as you can imagine, healing deep-seated tissue damage caused either by severe trauma or by many years of abnormal physical motion takes longer. Recovering from any severe injury or damage is like climbing a very tall mountain. As most experienced climbers will tell you, you don't climb a mountain all in one spurt. You climb for a while, then you rest. Sometimes you have camps set up at various points along the way so you can take a break and get acclimated to the altitude and weather conditions. If you're smart, you allocate plenty of time and carry plenty of supplies to support you in your journey to the summit.

The process of long-term healing is very similar. Let's say patients come into my office in acute pain. I'm not going to recommend they take up an exercise regimen right away, because even if exercise would benefit them, they're in too much pain to take that on. So I'll work with them to stabilize the subluxation first and begin to restore normal movement and functioning. It may take a few weeks for that to happen, depending on how much damage has been caused by the subluxation and how long it's been in place. After all, the tissues of the body have been conditioned to produce pain; now we're going to condition them to return to normal function, but it will take time. Once the body begins to remember how to function correctly, the pain will decrease or disappear, and then we can add things like exercises or an increase in daily activity; perhaps we can even address some other issues that have been raised by the initial subluxation. The journey from acute pain to health is accomplished over time, and is almost never straight line. Instead, it occurs in cycles and includes rest stops along the way, where the body can get used to a new way of moving or functioning before the next stage of healing begins.

In the kind of chiropractic work I do, which focuses on adjusting the upper neck area, I typically see patients go through very predictable cycles of healing, usually extending over a period of three months. While evidence of the existence of a three-month healing cycle is anecdotal, there is a physiological logic behind it. Different cells in the body renew themselves over different periods of time. For instance, most red blood cells live approximately 120 days. Skin cells renew themselves every three to six months. All the cells and tissues in the body replace themselves over predictable periods of time. When you treat healing as a natural occurrence (rather than one you artificially accelerate through introduction of a chemical called a drug), it makes sense that replacement of damaged cells with healthy ones would be tied to the cell's normal rate of renewal. So in this way, the natural birth, growth, and death of the cells within the body support the observed phenomenon of a three-month healing cycle.

What is less clearly explainable but also confirmed by observation of the process of healing is the phenomenon called *retracing*. Say you've been going through a tough time physically for a few years. You've had some pretty bad chest infections, perhaps a few digestive upsets, and also some major problems with your knees. Then you have an episode of back pain and decide to go to a chiropractor. The chiropractor starts you on a course of treatment designed to handle a number of subluxations of your spine. Your back pain gets better quickly—but over the next few weeks, as you continue your treatment plan, you notice some strange things starting to happen. One day you develop a little persistent cough for no reason. That goes away, and then you experience a little stomach sensitivity to certain foods. Then your knees start to ache as they haven't done in a few years. You report your symptoms to your chiropractor and say, "I'm not sure I should keep coming in—my back feels great, but the rest of me isn't so good!"

Your chiropractor then explains that we store memories of every "health event" within our nervous system and other tissues. When the body is finally allowed to let go of subluxations that have been affecting the spine for many years, sometimes old health problems linked to those subluxations begin to show up. What's happening is actually good: The body is releasing vestiges of those old illnesses, accidents, and traumas and returning to healthy, normal functioning. It's as if health is at the center of an onion, and to reach it we have to peel away layers of disease, trauma, and abnormal functioning.

Retracing also occurs with other alternative medical practices, such as acupuncture and homeopathy. This is not surprising, since all these practices are searching to help the body heal itself at the deepest possible level. To achieve that, you may have to be patient, allow the body to process change in its own good time, and be willing to be a little uncomfortable as the body releases residual traces of old illnesses and/or traumas. Only then can your core of radiant, natural, vital health be revealed.

▶ Using Chiropractic to Support Your Long-Term Health

One of the caveats you hear about chiropractors is that you're going to have to come back all the time. In reality, your length of treatment depends on what you want from your chiropractic care. If all you want is reduction of acute symptoms, then depending on the severity of your problem it could take anywhere from two to six visits spread over six to twelve weeks. That's how allopathic chiropractors treat patients: They give adjustments to treat an acute condition, and if the condition doesn't resolve in a certain period of time, then patients are referred to a conventional medical specialist, such as an orthopedist. But most chiropractors regard the elimination of symptoms as the easiest part of a course of treatment. Getting someone to feel good is only the basic outcome, one that may do very little to restore proper functioning of the spine and nervous system. If all that the chiropractor does is remove the pain and stop there, the chances of the condition recurring are much greater.

How long it will take to restore high-level functionality depends on the condition of the spine and the age of the patient. With a weeks-old baby, the spine is malleable and any damage has not been set in stone, so to speak, so one or two chiropractic adjustments (followed by ongoing preventive care) can restore functionality quickly. Older children or teenagers may take a few months of regular care to get the spine back to a healthy state. But with adults in their twenties, thirties, forties, or fifties, all too often the spine hasn't been functioning optimally for years. There may be considerable damage to the soft tissues surrounding the vertebrae, or maybe even deterioration in the bones due to improper movement. In these cases, it may take upward of a year or two to heal the damage fully and restore as much functionality to the spine as possible. With patients in their sixties and seventies, it can take even longer, and the outcome may not be as good due to the extent of the damage. But almost everyone can experience some increase in function with regular chiropractic care.

In the Introduction you met Shirley, who came into my office having suffered severe daily headaches for fifty years. I recommended she come in three times a week for three weeks, then twice a week for a while, and then we'd see how she was doing. Well, her headaches weren't gone after five or six visits—but they were 50 percent better after three months, and about 95 percent better after a year. It took only a few visits to correct the subluxations that were the cause of her headaches; however, her body needed time to adjust to a new level of functioning and to heal the damage done to the soft tissue surrounding her spine. Once the healing and realignment of her spine occurred, the headaches essentially went away. If she had stopped treatment at the fifth or sixth visit, however, the benefits she had attained might not have held, simply because the malfunction was so ingrained. Luckily, the patient believed in the benefit of chiropractic enough to stick with the program even though she wasn't experiencing the immediate relief she craved. Now she enjoys a headache-free life and gives all the credit to her chiropractic care.

Unfortunately, once a subluxation exists, there is some degree of permanent damage, because the scar tissue in the affected area will never be as good as the original tissue. That's why chiropractic maintenance throughout life is important. In most cases, I tell my patients that restoring proper function will require that I continue to monitor their spines for one to three years. The restoration process (returning the spine to its optimal level of functioning) usually requires visits about once a month or more. After patients reach their highest level of function (which probably will never be quite 100 percent, but is almost always much better than before they began care), most people go into maintenance care, with visits anywhere from once a month to once a quarter. Different chiropractors may recommend different schedules for maintenance care, but almost all of them stress the need for ongoing regular visits to maintain spine health.

Let's look at some typical problems that cause people to visit their chiropractors, and what you might expect from a course of care.

Back Pain

While there are many causes of back pain, frequently back pain arises from subluxation and subluxation related problems such as muscle spasm and abnormal joint mechanics, as described in Chapter 5. There may be inflammation created by the subluxation itself. In cases where the subluxation has been in place for a long time, or where there has been damage to the disk due to trauma, problems such as disk herniation and prolapse may occur.

For most back and neck pain, chiropractors will see patients three to five times a week for the first couple of weeks, then reduce the number of visits to once or twice a week for a few more weeks. This program of care usually lasts four to six weeks and is focused on helping patients feel better. Once this initial phase of short-term relief is completed, most chiropractors will recommend a second course of care designed to help avoid relapse, strengthen the spine, and restore proper function. Visits during the second course of care may be as frequent as two visits per week or as seldom as once every other week. This phase will continue for three to five months longer.

After completing relief and reconstruction care, many chiropractors will recommend chiropractic care for maintenance of your health. Maintenance care is care for life, and the recommended frequency of visits will range from twice a month to a checkup every three to six months. More commonly, the recommended maintenance level of care is once per month. The frequency of visits in the relief, reconstructive, and maintenance programs is determined by the overall health of your spine and the technical approach of the doctor.

When being treated for back pain, most patients will begin to feel better somewhere between the third and fifth adjustment. In a few cases, back pain can go away completely after just one adjustment, but this is the exception rather than the rule. If the pain does go away fairly quickly (in one to three visits), the problem is not really resolved. Restoration of normal joint mechanics and healing of local tissue and nerves can take months to complete even after the patient feels better. If the problem is extremely acute (as in a car accident) or there is long-term chronicity (as in arthritis), it may take a number of weeks and up to a few months for the back pain to show significant improvement. If your problem fits one of these categories, have patience with yourself and your chiropractor.

Disk problems in the neck or back can respond to chiropractic care as well, but treatment takes time. In some cases I have seen serious disk problems take over a year to become fixed and stable. In some cases where damage has progressed to the point where the body cannot heal itself, disk problems may need medical intervention to resolve. (Ideally, chiropractic care will begin long before the damage reaches this level. However, there are some studies indicating that conditions as severe as herniated or prolapsed disks can be helped with alternative treatments, including chiropractic. See Appendix I, "Conditions Helped by Chiropractic Care.")

William's wife brought him to my clinic, even though his expectations of "bone crackers," as he called chiropractors, were minimal. He had been experiencing debilitating lower back pain, which prevented him from driving, sitting, or standing for any period of time. An MRI exam had shown damage to the lower spine area, and the on-site surgeon had told him his only options were drugs and surgery.

In my initial workup, I discovered that William had three misaligned vertebrae in his neck, his shoulders were out of balance, and one of his legs was almost a half inch shorter than the other. I adjusted William on that first visit and ended up having to do three individual adjustments almost every visit. While William is still on the road to full recovery, his pain has almost completely resolved, he can sit, stand, and drive normally, and he says his day-to-day life is much better in general. More important, he was able to gain relief without drugs or surgery.

Another patient, Denise, was the mother of three young children: Lydia, intelligent, pretty, and proper; Dillon, inquisitive with a mix of seriousness and mischief; and Mallory, the youngest, a bright blond ball of energy. But Denise had no time for her kids because she was in too much pain. She had been under chiropractic care for most of her adult life, and it had helped her to manage recurring back and neck problems; but over the last year before coming to my office, her condition had worsened dramatically. In the last few weeks before I met her she was bedridden. Her low back pain was severe, with intense pain running down her right leg.

Her medical doctors had decided that Denise was a clear candidate for back surgery because of severe disk herniation. Her chiropractor, on the other hand, suggested that she try chiropractic one more time. Because of the unique approach used at my office, her chiropractor referred her to me, in spite of the fact that she lived three hours away.

When she came to my office, it took Denise twenty minutes to walk the fifteen steps from the curb to the front door, and literally almost thirty minutes to get from the front office to the back adjusting room. Watching her trying to walk was painful, as each step was an enormous exertion of effort and determination. You could see the grimace of pain in her face. But Denise was a strong woman—she should have been carried but insisted on walking.

Some three weeks into her course of care, she was still in significant pain but had improved almost 20 percent. By the time she had been under care for three months, her pain had reduced by almost 50 percent. Denise was very involved in her recovery, keeping a detailed graph of her pain level for the first nine months. The process of healing was slow, and her improvement in symptoms was up and down. But she stuck with the program, and by nine months into her care she had reached an almost pain-free state and was beginning to exercise again for the first time in over a year.

In a discussion we had some weeks into her treatment, Denise said that she and her husband, Morgan, thought it would be impossible for her to have any more children because of her severe back problems. I'm happy to report that their fourth child, Allison—the child who was not supposed to be—is now almost five years old. Allison is very mischievous like her brother, Dillon, and bright and energetic like her sisters. Denise and her family continue under maintenance chiropractic care because she decided to avoid surgery and take the long, difficult road to true health.

Headaches

Headaches have numerous causes, ranging from subluxation to brain tumors, although serious medical problems are the rare exception. This is why it is important to consider medical assessment for headache problems that don't resolve under chiropractic care. In reality, however, most patients with headaches come to the chiropractor as a last resort, after most medical and diagnostic approaches have already been tried.

Much research has shown that chiropractic care is effective for a variety of headaches—migraine, tension, cluster, cervicogenic (coming from the neck), and others. The course of care is usually much the same as the one described for back and neck pain, simply because the underlying cause of the headaches is also subluxation.

I have found that most headache problems resolve very quickly under chiropractic care, usually showing some relief after the first or second adjustment. With chronic headache problems, however, while an adjustment usually can offer some short-term relief, the most benefit is gained over the long run. As the neck subluxation heals and the tissues become healthier, chronic headache sufferers usually find that the frequency and intensity of headaches either decrease or disappear altogether.

Sharon was a young woman debilitated by headaches that lasted for days. She tried all manner of pain relievers, but they didn't even take the edge off her pain. Her course of treatment involved a series of adjustments to her neck, along with constant monitoring of her progress. (She told me that she was surprised I didn't adjust her at every visit, but I don't believe in adjusting when it's not necessary to support the body's return to normal function.) Sharon reports that her headaches have been almost eliminated, and she goes for weeks at a time without symptoms. "When I do have one, Dr. Lenarz knows exactly where and how to eliminate my pain," she said. I am confident that with continuing care, Sharon's headaches will be a thing of the past.

Numbness and Tingling

It is not uncommon to find that subluxation causes numbness and tingling in the arms, hands, fingers, legs, and feet. This is because nerves become unhealthy over time as a result of subluxation and begin to lose their normal function. Once again, there can be other causes of numbness aside from subluxation, but I have found that even in the case of neuropathy (inflammation and degeneration of peripheral nerves caused by diabetes or other problems) correction of subluxation can help these very intractable problems.

Numbness also can be caused by nerve interference in areas of the body other than the spine. Carpal tunnel syndrome (CTS) is an example. Some chiropractors treat CTS through adjustment of the wrists, physical therapy modalities, and bracing. As someone who specializes in upper cervical work, I have found that adjustment in the neck can reduce or eliminate CTS symptoms. (See also Appendix I.)

In any case, numbness and tingling are the signs of fairly advanced neurological breakdown and are not easily resolved. Once again, the course of care at a chiropractic office is primarily focused on subluxation correction, not specific treatment of the symptom. I find that numbness and tingling problems usually take many weeks to a few months of care to show significant improvement. It takes time for nerves to heal from this advanced state of damage. There is, of course, the occasional patient whose numbness and tingling problems disappear after just one or a few adjustments, but most people with this sort of problem need to be patient and allow time for healing.

Linda came to my clinic with a whole menu of problems: lower back pain that kept her from sleeping more than four or five hours at a time, fatigue (not surprising), and a pins-and-needles sensation in her arms and legs. She was surprised when I said I would work on her neck, and even more surprised when she didn't even feel the adjustments I gave her. But she was delighted with the results of her care. Her back pain disappeared, as did her pins and needles. Because she was able to sleep soundly, her fatigue diminished. Her health is improving all the time, she says, and adds, "I would have gone to a chiropractor a long time ago if I knew then what I know now!"

Digestive, Cardiovascular, Sinus, and Other Target Organs and Tissues

As discussed throughout this book, the nerves that come from the spine go to virtually all the cells, tissues, and organs in the body. Although chiropractic is not a cure-all for every health problem, nerve interference from subluxation potentially can affect any tissue in the body, leading to health problems in that area. Whether the health problem is acid reflux, problems with proper elimination, or overly sensitive sinuses that are subject to infection and allergic response, when the nerves to these target tissues are free of subluxation, the tissues become healthier. In most cases, the healing process follows a logical sequence. Once the subluxation is corrected, the local tissues near the spine begin to heal first. Then the nerves begin to heal, and then the target organs fed by those nerves can begin to regain their health.

However, just as the process of disease usually takes time to gain momentum, the process of returning to health takes time as well. That is because true health comes from the body repairing and replacing tissues and cells, and this process *must* take place over time.

For problems that are distant from the spine, or for target tissue ailments, the course of care may be similar to that of a person suffering from back pain: an initial course of relief care, followed by reconstructive and then maintenance care. The amount of time that it takes to feel better will be determined by the patient's age and the amount of tissue damage sustained before care begins. Some people have unexpectedly quick relief from their health problems; others will take longer to heal.

Lawrence, a young father, was having trouble keeping up with his toddler son. He came to my clinic hoping to eliminate the neck and back pain he experienced whenever he held his head in one position—to read or wash dishes, for example. He also revealed he was having hearing problems, he had problems waking because his balance was off, he couldn't concentrate, and he had difficulty digesting his food. Lawrence was lucky: His neck pain resolved fairly quickly. His other problems took a little longer to treat. Today he reports a 90 percent improvement in hearing, concentration, and digestion, and attributes a greater level of success in his career to the fact that he is so much healthier.

▶ The Chiropractic Lifestyle

Chiropractic care isn't a quick fix, although it can eliminate pain fairly quickly. Ideally it should be a lifestyle choice, in the same way you choose to eat a healthy diet or exercise. I liken chiropractic care to sessions with a physical trainer. When you start exercising under the guidance of a physical trainer you need to work with him or her several times a week so you can set patterns for proper physiological function. Once you have those patterns in place, then you can check in with your trainer once a month or once a quarter to get a new set of exercises based on your current level of functioning. But when you get to a certain level of physical performance, does that mean you don't have to exercise the rest of your life? No. If you eat well for a few months, does that mean you can eat whatever you like for the rest of your life and it doesn't matter? No. You have to continue exercising and eating well if you want to be healthy. And chiropractic care is just as vital a part of a healthy lifestyle as exercise and nutrition. In the same way you need to take care of your muscular and circulatory system through regular exercise, and your digestive system through proper nutritional habits, you need to take care of your nervous system through regular chiropractic care.

In the next few chapters we'll discuss some specific ways you can support your overall health and your chiropractic care through exercise, nutrition, stress reduction, and a long-term commitment to taking care of your body.

8

Using Exercise to Increase Your Energy and Support Your Health

When I was nine years old and my brother Pat was ten, we moved to Bloomfield Hills, Michigan, and made friends with a kid named Mike McAnn. I liked Mike. He had a quality that made us feel like something exciting was about to happen, that we all had something up our sleeves. Mike introduced my brother and me to the guilty pleasures of smoking. He'd steal cigarettes from his parents, and we would go into the fields next to our neighborhood, hide in a grove of trees, and puff away. It was bad and it was fun. I toyed with smoking off and on until I was about fourteen, and then I took it up seriously. It wasn't until I was thirty-five that I finally kicked the habit once and for all—and that was four years *after* I graduated from chiropractic school. I am living proof that even after you learn the fundamental principles of chiropractic, it can still take time to apply them.

Almost every choice we make in life leads us down one path or another. In terms of our health, the choices we make—about diet, exercise, handling stress, even how we choose to view our bodies—will increase, decrease, or maintain our level of well-being and vitality. If you're reading this book, it's pretty safe to assume that you're interested in making choices that will increase your experience of health. After all, the fundamental basis of chiropractic philosophy is the choice to regard health as a state of being where Innate Intelligence is allowed to flow freely, and the goal of health care as simply to restore the body's optimal function by removing blocks to that energy's flow.

But blocks are not caused just by trauma, or even by normal wear and tear. All too often they're the result of what the popular press calls "lifestyle choices"—like my choosing to smoke even though I knew it was bad for my health. Like choosing to eat unhealthful foods in copious quantities. Like choosing to sit around and watch TV instead of getting the exercise your body needs to stay fit. Like choosing to take a pill to get rid of a symptom instead of getting regular chiropractic or other health care to eliminate the cause of your discomfort. The lifestyle choices we make every single day have a far greater impact on our overall health than any treatment offered by any health care practitioner. But because healthy choices are often so simple to make yet so difficult to maintain, we tend to avoid them—until the damage to our health has gotten so great that we are forced either to seek treatment, change our ways, or both.

I have had numerous patients tell me that they were unlucky because they "caught" or "came down with" a certain disease or illness. Although there are always factors that we cannot control, such as genetics or toxins in our environment, chiropractic teaches us that we are *not* victims of diseases that "attack" us. It teaches that health and disease come from within, and health is the natural result of life being fully expressed. This has led me to believe strongly in the idea of responsibility. Not the kind that causes me to blame myself or feel guilty when I become sick, but one that allows me to recognize that I have choices to make—and that what I choose can play a powerful role in the creation of my own health.

In the early 1900s, chiropractors already were talking about the impact of lifestyle choices on our overall health, only the term they used was "survival values." The idea goes something like this: All the things you do, all of the activities you partake in, will either increase or decrease your chances of survival. Things that are bad for your health, like smoking a pack of cigarettes daily, have a negative survival value. Conversely, healthy actions, such as eating a balanced diet or walking two miles a day, would have a positive survival value. Chiropractic care has a positive survival value because it helps the body to function at a higher level of efficiency, allowing us to adapt better to our environment. We can assign a survival value to every thought we think and every choice we make. Most of the choices that we know are good for us, like eating healthy foods and exercising, have a positive survival value. But if you are like me, you've probably found that it is easier to *talk* about living a healthier life than it is to actually *do* it.

I have found a simple approach to this dilemma: I call it "baby steps." Instead of trying to change everything at once (which is often the way we try to do things), you take just one small baby step at a time. That way you can keep building on small successes until you actually achieve a lifestyle change. For instance, when I finally decided to quit smoking, I didn't try to give up cigarettes, start an exercise program, clean up my diet, begin relaxation exercises, and change my way of thinking all at once. For me, as for most of us, this would have been a formula for failure. Instead, I focused solely on eliminating cigarettes from my life. I didn't worry about my diet, I didn't focus on exercising, I didn't increase the time I spent meditating (although as I went through the cravings and withdrawal, I did find I could use diet, exercise, and meditation to support my efforts to quit). Taking lifestyle changes one baby step at a time allowed me to rebuild my health in a realistic and achievable way.

In Chapter 3 I talked about the law of entropy, which states that everything eventually settles into its state of lowest energy. Pyramids crumble, houses eventually fall, rocks turn to dust, even stars burn out. In other words, everything breaks down. But while this is true of living things as well, life fools entropy. Even though we know we can't live forever, for a brief period of time life actually grows, builds itself up, adapts to its environment, and defies the universal forces of entropy. This is life's magic. And unlike buildings, rocks, and stars, life has created another clever method to trick entropy—procreation. Life creates new life!

The ability to adapt, to hold at bay the forces that are always trying to tear us down, is the essence of our ability to stay healthy. The forces that reside within us, directed by Innate Intelligence, defend us against the forces that are constantly trying to break us down. This is the dance of life. Positive survival values are simply those things that tip the scale in our favor, in the direction of life and health.

▶ The Benefits of Exercise

How do we know we are healthy? We feel good, yes—but we also feel that our bodies are functioning at an optimal level. We can move in many different ways without pain or difficulty. We breathe fully; we have the strength to take on our daily tasks. We sleep deeply and digest our food easily and well. We adapt to our surroundings and to the stresses and strains of everyday life with ease. To maintain health, all the systems of our bodies must be functioning properly. And one of the best ways to increase our level of function is with regular exercise.

I'm sure you've read over and over again about the benefits of aerobic exercise to your cardiovascular system, and how weight training can increase muscle tone and even bone density (a special concern for women as they age). You've probably heard how exercise can improve digestion, elimination, respiration, and lymph flow, and increase the efficiency of almost every single organ in the body. So I'm not going to focus on any of those well-proven results. Instead, I want to talk about how certain forms of exercise can provide some surprising benefits to the health and functioning of your central nervous system.

As I said in Chapter 5, the spinal cord is surrounded by the vertebrae, which are supported by a complex interrelated system of soft tissues, including cartilage, muscles, ligaments, and tendons. Now, like all muscles, those surrounding and supporting the spine (many of which are grouped under the term *postural muscles*) can become weakened through disuse or strained through misuse. If you've ever had the unpleasant experience of pulling a muscle in your back, you know what I mean!

It used to be that if someone complained of back pain, the recommended course of treatment was complete bed rest for several weeks. This prescription has been completely reversed in recent years, as evidence has continued to mount that mild exercise helps to reduce the chronicity (that is, the severity and recurrence) of back pain in most patients. Even conventional medical doctors now agree that patients with back pain should be encouraged to keep moving and even do some gentle exercise as quickly as possible.

Chiropractors have long been interested in the effect of exercise on back pain, and there have been numerous studies done on the effectiveness of exercise, spinal adjustment, or a combination of the two in eliminating back pain and restoring health. Researchers have found that the right kind of exercise combined with a regular program of spinal adjustment is the most effective treatment for restoring optimal functioning to the body, far exceeding the results of exercise or adjustment alone.

When I have a patient with acute pain, I'm not going to give him or her exercises right away. First we need to stabilize the subluxation and get the muscles moving properly again. Once the soft tissue surrounding the vertebrae has had a chance to heal (see Chapter 5) and things are relatively stable again—and the patient is out of acute pain—then I suggest the introduction of some functional exercises or increasing the activity level. Remember, chiropractic care is about restoring the fullest range of motion possible, and the only way to do that is for the muscles themselves to support the vertebrae as they twist and turn.

By the way, if someone has pain in the lower back, he or she usually thinks it's a result of weak abdominal muscles. But research has shown that the muscles in the front of the stomach have very little to do with chronic back pain. With chronic back pain, the muscles that are the most involved are the extensors—the ones that make us arch our back backward. So again, the cure for back pain is to build and strengthen the muscles that support the back and spine.

To provide the spine with adequate support, we need to make sure our postural muscles are strong. How do we do this? By the proper forms of exercise. Weightlifting exercises like those you do in a gym are excellent for building muscles in general. However, our postural muscles need not only to bear weight but also to move freely and fully. Strength *plus* flexibility is the goal. And weight-bearing exercises don't necessarily provide the correct kind of stretching and moving required to promote flexibility of the back. Luckily, there are a couple of forms of exercise that are great for both flexibility and strength of those postural muscles. Specifically, I like to recommend hatha yoga and tai chi to my patients.

The benefits of hatha yoga and tai chi go beyond just flexibility and strength, however. In Chapter 4, I talked about the information our nerves transmit to the spinal cord and brain. A large part of this information is sensory data—what we see, hear, feel, taste, touch, and smell. But we have a couple of other senses that are less commonly known, and one that is very important to our overall health is our sense of balance or *proprioception,* which tells us where our bodies are oriented in space and how we are moving. If our sense of proprioception is off, we can lose our balance and fall more easily. Infants and very young children don't have very good proprioception; it takes a while for them to develop a sense of where they are in space and how their muscles function. And we often see deterioration in proprioception as people age, which is one of the reasons old people lose their balance and fall more frequently. Because it improves the communication between the brain and body, regular chiropractic care actually improves proprioception in many people. Many kinds of exercise are also beneficial in improving proprioception, balance, and coordination, but few are more effective than yoga and tai chi.

Why? Both systems of exercise focus on balancing the body as it moves into and out of certain postures. The physical principle involved is called *co-activation of muscles.* When you go into and out of yoga postures, or flow through the sequence of movements of a tai chi exercise routine, you're using all sorts of different muscle groups at the same time. The muscles on both sides of the body are activated equally, and in conjunction with many other groups of muscles. This creates an ideal integration of muscle and balance function to support the health of the body in general, and the spine in particular. Making yoga or tai chi a regular part of your fitness routine will improve your balance and coordination, cause your muscles to work together smoothly, and stretch your spine and the supporting muscles through their range of motion, allowing them to maintain optimal functioning.

▶ Developing Flexibility and Strength Through Hatha Yoga

You may have seen a lot of press lately about many different kinds and schools of yoga—Iyenegar, Kundalini, Ashtanga, and so on—but they all are variations within the overall category of hatha yoga. Hatha yoga was developed thousands of years ago in India. It is a system of exercise, breathing, and mental focus designed to keep body, mind, and spirit as healthy as possible from childhood to old age. Properly done, these exercises are designed to build strength and flexibility into muscles, improve range of motion, promote overall joint health, and encourage relaxation.

We'll look first at a series of basic yoga postures and movements. If you are just beginning an exercise program, a simple ten- to fifteen-minute yoga routine is a great place to start, as it gets you used to breathing deeper, and moving more fully and easily than you may have done before. If you are already working out, chances are you can benefit from paying more attention to proper stretching and range-of-motion exercises. Even if you already incorporate stretching in your workout, I encourage you to consider adding some of these exercises, to gain their balance and muscle co-activation benefits. (As always, if you are suffering from back or neck problems, please discuss these exercises with your chiropractor before proceeding.)

These yoga exercises will be presented in two parts. The first part will outline a basic ten- to fifteen-minute routine, which is done sitting or lying on the floor. These exercises primarily focus on the legs, pelvis, and lower back, and are designed to improve range of motion and increase flexibility. Even if you've never exercised before, these poses are safe because they keep the pelvis stabilized, thereby promoting a healthy, nontaxing stretch. The second set of exercises is more advanced and includes a number of standing postures designed to develop better posture, improve balance, and strengthen muscles. The full routine (both sets) takes between thirty and forty-five minutes, depending on your speed and the number of repetitions of each posture.

Remember to take baby steps. You can begin with just one or two exercises, or with the least amount of time or repetitions per posture. The important thing is to get started right away and be consistent. Whatever part of the routine you choose, I recommend that you start with a minimum of three days a week and build up to five times per week.

Proper Breathing

In our rushed and anxious world, we tend to breathe very shallowly—we don't use our full lungs. We often hold our breath without even knowing it. If you pay close attention, you will find that whenever you're experiencing pain, anxiety, anger, or another negative emotion, you tend to either hold your breath or breathe very quickly and shallowly. Although this may have some value in the fight-or-flight response (we need to breathe quickly when we're running away from danger), when we are chronically in this state our body is robbed of oxygen.

Every cell in our body needs to "breathe." Every cell takes in oxygen, which is used to create energy for the cell to do its work, and expels a waste product, carbon dioxide. How does the oxygen get to the cells in our body? A simple yet miraculous process. When we breathe in, the air goes into our lungs. There the oxygen molecules are picked up by the hemoglobin in our red blood cells and transported to every cell throughout the body. The hemoglobin also picks up the carbon dioxide waste product from the cells and transports it back to the lungs, where it is exhaled with our outgoing breath. Essentially our lungs act as a giant train station, where the oxygen "train" goes out to the rest of the body and the carbon dioxide "train" comes in.

When we breathe shallowly, we are both depriving our body of oxygen and not efficiently throwing off the carbon dioxide. Not good! When we breathe fully, however, the hemoglobin molecules leave the lungs filled with as much oxygen as they can carry. They can also eliminate more carbon dioxide on the return trip. So proper breathing is not only helpful for these exercises, it's good for life.

All yoga exercises are based on proper breathing technique. Breathing correctly will allow you to relax; it will increase your energy and help you avoid injury. Because each of the following exercises is paced according to specific breathing patterns, we will start by building our base with the *full yoga breath*.

LEARNING THE FULL YOGA BREATH

1. Start by paying attention to your breathing. Sitting in a chair or cross-legged on the floor, take a few moments and do that now. Usually when we pay attention to our breath, it automatically begins to slow down and deepen. Now pay closer attention. You will probably notice that you are using only about the top one-quarter to one-third of your lungs.

2. Now, take a *really deep* breath. If you are like most of us, what you will notice is that your chest rises when you do this. However, our goal with the yoga breath is to have the *abdomen* rise, followed by the chest expanding.

3. A good way to practice this is to lie on the floor and put a book on your stomach. Take a deep breath and see if you can make the book rise—not just by pushing your stomach up, but by breathing deep down into your lungs so that the abdomen automatically rises. When you breathe out, empty your lungs all the way—give an extra, gentle push at the end of your exhale to let that carbon dioxide out of your body. Continue to work with this practice until you find it natural to fill your lungs and raise your abdomen.

4. Next, practice a full breath while sitting and/or standing. Roll your shoulders back gently so that they are not slouching forward and closing down your chest. Think of your lungs as a pitcher: As you breathe in, fill the pitcher starting with the bottom. The inhale should first fill the bottom of your

lungs, and then rise progressively to fill the top of your lungs. As you breathe out, visualize emptying the pitcher in the opposite order. The exhale should first empty the top of the lungs, then the middle, and finally the bottom. The breath should be slow, steady, and even, not hurried or anxious. A complete yoga breath is one full inhale and one full exhale.

5. Once you have the mechanics of the yoga breath down, practice doing ten breaths in a row. Pay attention, making sure that each breath is slow and deliberate, and don't hyperventilate.

Unless otherwise noted, the full yoga breath should be employed with all the exercises described in this chapter. But you don't have to limit this breathing technique to just exercise time. The full yoga breath is good to do when you are tired, anxious, stressed, or angry, as it will help energize and calm you. Anytime that we pay attention to our breath, slow it down, and breathe deeply, it can help us to relax and generate a greater sense of well-being.

General Points

It is probably best to do your yoga exercises first thing in the morning or last thing in the evening. You will find that you will be more flexible in the evening and stiffer in the morning. I enjoy doing my exercises first thing in the morning. It sets the tone for a relaxing day and helps me feel more comfortable and energetic. You will want to avoid eating for one to three hours before doing these exercises. It is also best to empty your bladder and bowels before beginning.

If possible, find a space where you won't be disturbed. The floor should be somewhat cushioned with a carpet or rug. If done on a hard floor, you should use an exercise mat. To help prevent injuries and ensure maximum stretch, your exercise surface should be nonskid. It's also usually best to do these postures in your bare feet.

With yoga exercises, proper form will increase the benefits you experience from each stretch. Please refer to the photos illustrating each posture if you have any questions. When first beginning your yoga exercises, you might want to check your posture in a mirror to make sure you're holding the stretch properly. And as with any exercise, if you experience major discomfort during any stretch, release the posture immediately, and then check with your chiropractor or other health care provider.

Exercises While Sitting or Lying on the Floor

BASIC STRETCH

This exercise is very simple and a good place to start your exercise routine. It will help you begin your exercises by relaxing first.

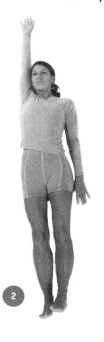

1. Lie down on your back with your arms comfortably at your side, with your feet and legs far enough apart that they are relaxed.

2. As you breathe in slowly, raise your right arm above your head so that your bicep is next to your ear. Reach back until you feel the muscles in your arm stretching. At the same time, stretch your right leg by pulling it downward, in the opposite direction to your arm. Stretch from your heel, not your toes; imagine you have a cord coming from your right heel that is pulling your leg as if to lengthen it. You should feel stretching all along the right side of the body, and a sense of traction on the

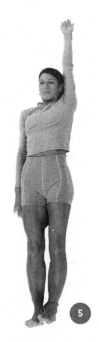

right side of the back. Inhale as you slowly and gently stretch. When you begin to exhale, bring your arm back to your side and let the leg relax.

3. Repeat with the left arm and leg. Remember to breathe slowly and stretch gently. In most of the exercises, if you focus on moving unhurriedly, with precision, and in unison with proper breathing, you will avoid overstretching and pulling the muscles.

4. Next, bring the right arm up over your head while lengthening the left leg by stretching from the left heel. This is a crisscross stretch. You should feel traction along the spine, stretching the mid- and lower back areas.

5. Next, stretch the left arm up while pulling down with the right heel.

6. Finally, stretch both arms above your head while stretching and lengthening both legs. Perform this stretch one to three times.

VARIED LEG STRETCH

This exercise consists of three separate stretches for each leg. If you have knee problems or if this exercise causes knee pain, don't do it. Yoga should bring you to the limit of your flexibility and perhaps slightly beyond, but it should not be painful.

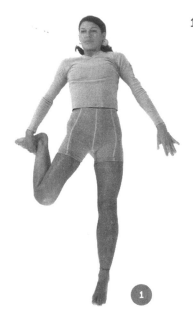

1. While continuing to lie on your back, inhale and bend your right knee as if trying to fold the leg under you, but instead, bring your right foot out and away from your body to rest next to your right hip. Your knee should be pointing down and slightly to the right. Your hip should lift slightly off the floor, and the tension on the front of your right thigh should hold the knee slightly above the floor. You should feel stretching along the front of your thigh, from the knee to the groin. If you do not feel stretching in this area, bring the foot farther away from your body (still resting it on the floor) and more toward your head until you do. Once you feel the stretching, hold for one to three full yoga breaths.

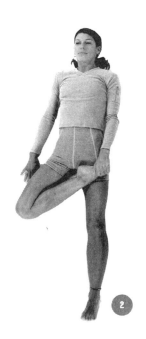

2. While exhaling, bring the right foot back around, bending the knee in the opposite direction, so that the right heel comes to rest on top of the left thigh, just below the groin. The right knee should be pointing away from your body toward the right. Use your leg muscles to pull the knee gently down toward the floor. (It may not be necessary to increase this stretch by pulling your knee down if you already feel significant stretching just by putting your leg in this position.) The stretch should be felt on the inside of the thigh. Hold this position for one to two full yoga breaths. Relax the leg while inhaling, then increase the stretch while exhaling.

3. While inhaling, unfold the right leg and bring it flat on the floor next to the left leg. Exhale and hold. On the next inhale, lift the right leg up so that the heel is pointing straight into the air. Grasp the leg with both hands just below the knee, and use your hands to gently pull the leg toward your chest, stretching the muscles in the back of the thigh. If possible, keep your leg straight; don't bend the knee. The foot should be flexed (toes pointing toward your body). As you exhale, bring the right leg back to the floor in the neutral position.

4. Take one full yoga breath, and then repeat all three steps with the other leg.

BOUNCING LEGS

Most of the stretching done in yoga does *not* include bouncing. This exercise is a rare exception.

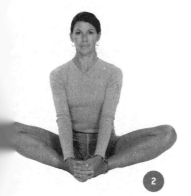

1. Come into a sitting position, with your legs flat on the floor in front of you. Your back should be kept as straight as is comfortably possible.

2. While inhaling, bring your feet in toward your groin, with the bottoms of your feet flat against one another. Grasp your feet with your hands. Your knees should be pointing outward.

3. Continuing to breathe slowly and evenly, gently bounce your knees up and down, feeling the stretch close to the groin. Do this for one to three minutes.

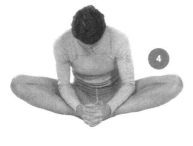

4. While exhaling, bend forward and pull your chest toward your feet. Let your elbows move in front of the legs and allow your back to bend (curve) forward. You should feel a significant stretching along the whole back, into the buttock and in the inner thighs. Take one to two breaths in this position, using your hands to pull your chest down toward your feet while exhaling, releasing the tension slightly while inhaling.

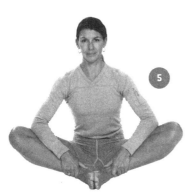

5. On the next exhale, grasp each ankle with the corresponding hand (right hand grasps the right ankle, left grasps left) and rest your elbows on the inside of your knees. Push down gently. You are using your arms as levers to increase the stretch of the inner thigh. Release while inhaling.

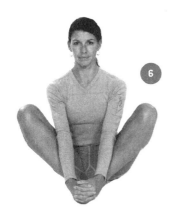

6. Exhale, grasp your feet again, and pull your knees inward and upward to press gently against your arms.

HAMSTRING STRETCH

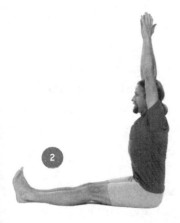

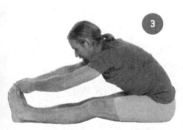

1. In a sitting position, bring your legs together in front of you, and sit with as straight a back as possible while being comfortable.

2. Inhale, and reach your arms above your head. Clasp your hands together, stretching upward.

3. As you exhale, bend forward from the waist and bring your arms down and forward toward your feet. Your ankles should be flexed, as if you were trying to point your toes back toward your head. If you can reach your toes, do so. If you cannot, your hands should come to rest on your calves or thighs. It is important to keep your back straight; don't curve your back as you bend forward. The object is not to see if you can bring your chest against your thighs, but to stretch the back of your legs and buttock. Hold for one full yoga breath.

4. As you inhale slowly, come back to the sitting position and bring your arms over your head again. Repeat this cycle at least three times.

LEGS, BACK, AND SIDE STRETCH

1. From the sitting position, with your legs straight out in front of you, inhale as you spread your legs apart as much as possible. Your legs should form a V. Spread your legs until you feel that they are as far apart as possible without causing spasm or injury.

2. Keeping your back straight, bend forward slowly as you reach your arms out in front of you and exhale, feeling your inner thighs, lower back, and hips stretch.

3. As you inhale, come back to the sitting position. Exhale slowly.

4. Bring your left arm in an arching motion over your head as you inhale. Then begin to bend your body sideways and slightly forward toward the right leg as you exhale, bringing your left arm over your head as if trying to reach for the right foot. Your ribs on your right side are being pulled toward your right thigh, and you ought to feel stretching and opening of the ribs on the left side. Hold your right ankle or foot gently with your right hand. The foot should be flexed. If you can't reach your ankle or foot, grab hold of your calf.

5. Inhale as you straighten to the sitting position.

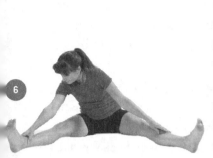

6. Now you are going to stretch toward the right leg again but from a slightly different angle. Instead of bending sideways, turn your body from the waist toward your right leg and then bend forward, bringing your chest toward your thigh as you exhale. Bring your arms forward and, if possible, grasp your ankle. You can use your arms to pull yourself slightly downward, but make sure to keep your back straight and to stretch slowly and carefully.

7. Inhale as you come back up to the sitting position, facing forward.

8. Repeat steps 1 through 7 to the right side, bringing your right arm over your head. Stretch both sides a minimum of three times each.

CAT STRETCH

Up to this point, all of our exercises have involved either lying down or sitting. Now we are going to move into some other basic positions.

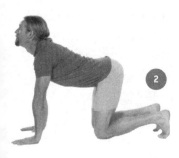

1. The Cat Stretch begins on your hands and knees. Your arms and legs are shoulder width apart and pointing straight down, 90 degrees to the floor. Your head is held in a neutral position, your eyes looking down at the floor. Your ankles are flexed and your toes are tucked under.

2. Inhale as you tilt your pelvis down toward the floor and arch your lower back forward, pulling it and your abdomen toward the floor. As you

continue to inhale, arch the midback in the same direction, as if trying to form your back into a C shape, with the open end of the C pointing up. Don't bend your arms or legs. Continue this arching by lifting the head up as if trying to look overhead. The arching of the neck should form a continuous, smooth line with the midback. Don't overextend the neck! (Overextending the neck could cause problems in the upper neck.) Inhale the entire time that you stretch.

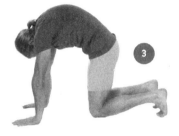

3. As you exhale, reverse the curve of the back, starting again with the lower back. Tilt the pelvis up, pulling the back and abdomen up toward the sky. Then arch the midback up, like a cat. Tilt the head forward and tuck the chin toward the chest. Now the C shape has its open side toward the floor. This exercise should proceed as slowly as your breathing will allow. Think of the motion of the spine as a wave, starting from the lower back and moving up through the neck.

4. Perform the cycle three to six times.

This completes the first set of recommended exercises. If you wish, you can add some of the following postures to your routine even before you are doing all of the sitting or lying postures. However, I do recommend that you include at least a few of the first set as part of your regular practice, as they will prepare your body for the more rigorous standing postures described next.

Moving into Standing Postures

These postures are designed to build on the balance and muscle strength you have developed by doing the seated or lying stretches in the first set. Continue to practice body awareness as you do these exercises; you want to give your muscles a good stretch but not overextend. A little discomfort is fine, but pain or a feeling that your muscles are pulling past a healthful stretch is not. Like the first set of exercises, this group should take you around ten to fifteen minutes to complete.

DOWNWARD-FACING DOG

This posture resembles a dog stretching, thus the name.

1. Begin on your hands and knees. Your legs should be shoulder width apart, with your knees directly below your hips. Your arms should also be shoulder width apart and slightly forward of your shoulders. Your head should be held in a neutral position, looking down at the floor. Your ankles should be flexed, and your toes tucked under.

2. While exhaling, straighten your legs and raise your buttocks toward the ceiling. You should be bending at the hips, with your legs straight. Do not bend your knees. The spine should be elongated, not curved.

3. Once the buttocks are lifted, try to gently pull your heels down toward the floor. Attempt to hold this posture for three to five breaths.

4. If this posture isn't too strenuous, you can add a further stretch by gently attempting to lower your head inward, toward your feet, as if to place the crown of your head on the floor. This is an advanced pose but will provide additional benefit for the mid- and upper back.

This exercise requires flexibility in the hamstrings, so you may need to practice the Hamstring Stretch (see page 133) along with a number of the first set of exercises for a while before moving into Downward-Facing Dog.

MOUNTAIN POSE

This is a deceptively easy posture, but it has very powerful benefits. It forms the basis for proper standing posture and for more advanced yoga exercises. If you can master this pose, it will be of unending bene-fit to the health of your spine. You will need to pay close attention to every aspect of how you stand. We'll start from the feet and work our way up.

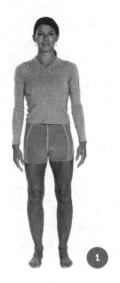

1. Stand erect with your bare feel parallel, about three to five inches apart. Your feet ought to be as flat against the floor as possible, with your toes spread apart and pointing straight ahead. Your weight should be evenly distributed between your feet. Do not lean forward onto the balls of your feet or backward onto the heels. Relax your toes if you feel as if they are trying to grasp the floor.

2. Tighten the muscles on the front of your thighs, as if using them to lift up your kneecaps. Next, contract the muscles on the back of the thighs and tighten your buttocks muscles. This will tend to pull your sacrum (tailbone) slightly forward. This stabilizes and balances the pelvic girdle. (We will refer to this part of the stance as "activating your legs" in other postures.) It is important to avoid overextending or locking the knees. They should not arch backward, but should remain straight. It may be useful to have a mirror to see if your legs are straight from the side view. Your legs should also be parallel.

3. If your knees tend to point in or out, perform the following movement: Inhale, and then while exhaling, bend your knees slightly. Keep your knees pointing forward as much as possible. Do this by keeping your legs parallel and your weight evenly distributed on both feet. Then, while inhaling, slowly unbend the knees, coming back to a straight leg position. As you straighten your knees, pay close attention to keeping your legs parallel and avoiding overextension. As you come

back into the straight leg position, you are activating the same muscles that I described a moment ago, to stand erect and stabilize the pelvis. *Although your legs and knees are straight, do not lock your knees.*

4. The stomach should be held in gently.

5. The chest should be held forward by making sure the shoulders are erect and slightly back, not rounded. To bring your shoulders into the proper position, roll your shoulders up and back and then let them relax, with your arms dangling slightly behind your chest.

6. Your spine should feel like it is being stretched upward, with the neck and head held erect. You might like to visualize a string tied to the top of your head, pulling your head and spine up gently into a vertical posture.

7. Once in position, hold for a minimum of one minute and a maximum of three. Remember to keep the leg muscles activated and use the full yoga breath throughout.

TRIANGLE POSE

You may want to have a sturdy table, railing, or kitchen counter behind you for support as you move into Triangle Pose.

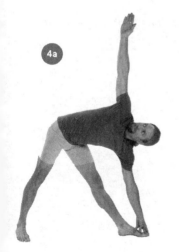

1. Begin with Mountain Pose. Activate your legs as described in step 2 above in Mountain Pose, then step your feet apart about three to four feet.

2. Turn your right foot out so that the heel is pointing back toward the arch of the left foot. (This creates a 90-degree angle with the left foot.) Then turn the left foot in about 15 degrees from its original position.

3. Inhale as you raise your arms slowly away from your sides, bringing them parallel to the floor, palms pointing down. Exhale and lengthen your spine, using the imagery of the string pulling up from the top of your head.

4. Inhale again, and while exhaling, reach your right hand out over your right leg, allowing yourself to bend slightly at the hips (not the waist). Keep your arms pointing straight out from your body as you reach your right hand toward the floor. Your right hand should come to rest on the floor behind your right foot. If you

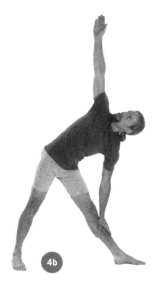

4b

can't reach that far (most people can't until they've been practicing this pose for a while), grasp the right ankle or leg. If reaching to the leg or floor is too strenuous, you can rest your right elbow on the table or railing for support.

5. The left arm should be pointing straight up, maintaining its 90-degree angle to the body. The natural tendency is to allow the body and left arm to bend forward, so you may need to focus on pulling the left arm and shoulder back. This keeps the left arm pointing straight up and the body bending sideways.

6. Hold this position for thirty to sixty seconds, breathing normally.

7. Inhale as you rise from this position to standing, with arms still held straight out at your sides and palms toward the floor. Repeat to the left.

8. Perform this movement one to three times to each side.

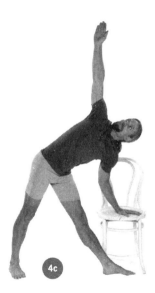

4c

WARRIOR POSE

As in the last pose, you may want to have a sturdy table, railing, or counter behind you.

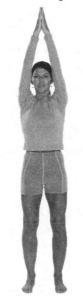

1. Begin with Mountain Pose. Inhale and lift your arms straight out from your body, raising your arms above your head, joining your palms together.

2. Exhale, and then while inhaling, stretch your arms up, reaching for the sky, palms still together. If you can maintain your balance, rise onto your toes while stretching.

3. While exhaling, come down off your toes and bring your arms back down until they are at a 90-degree angle to the body, parallel with the floor, and palms facing downward. Make sure your legs are still activated.

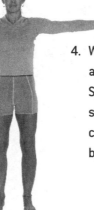

4. While inhaling, step your legs four to five feet apart depending on how flexible and tall you are. Spread your legs to the point where you feel stretching but no pain. If needed, at this point you can use the table or counter to stabilize yourself by bringing your arms down to rest on the support.

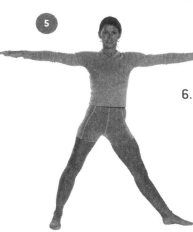

5. Exhale, and then while inhaling turn your right foot out 90 degrees to your stance, and the left foot in 15 degrees (as you did in Triangle Pose).

6. Exhale while turning your head to the right and bending the right knee until it is exactly over the right ankle. Do not flex the right knee beyond the ankle. Keep the left leg straight and activated. Remember to keep your spine erect with your arms extended and stretched, as if someone were pulling on each arm.

7. Hold this pose for ten to sixty seconds, breathing in a relaxed manner.

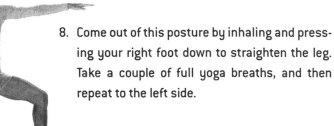

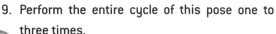

8. Come out of this posture by inhaling and pressing your right foot down to straighten the leg. Take a couple of full yoga breaths, and then repeat to the left side.

9. Perform the entire cycle of this pose one to three times.

UPPER BACK, SHOULDER, AND CHEST STRETCH

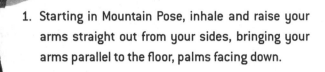

1. Starting in Mountain Pose, inhale and raise your arms straight out from your sides, bringing your arms parallel to the floor, palms facing down.

2. While exhaling, slowly and gently swing your arms forward, bending at a 90-degree angle at the elbows. Bring your left arm so that the elbow is directly in front of your chest and the arm is parallel to the floor, palm facing down. The right elbow should come to rest on top of the left arm, with the forearm pointing upward and the palm facing the left.

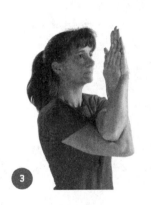

3. Next, reach the left arm back toward the right arm, entwining the arms so that the left palm comes together with the right one. If your hands cannot reach each other, use a sock or small towel that you can hold with your right hand and grasp with your left.

4. Hold this position for two to three breaths. When inhaling, lift your entwined arms upward toward the sky. You should feel stretching in the midback area. While exhaling, allow the arms and shoulders to relax while still maintaining the posture. Keep your head level and your legs activated.

5. On exhaling, unlock your arms and gently swing them back out, away from your sides, bringing them parallel to the floor once again, palms facing downward.

6. Inhale, and then while exhaling, bring your arms in front of you once again, this time with the left arm on top of the right. Repeat the pose in this position for the same number of breaths as the first part. Once you have completed the sequence, bring your arms out, away from your sides once again, while you exhale.

7. Inhale, and then while exhaling, bring your arms behind you and allow your hands to grasp one another with interlacing fingers. Your arms should be relaxed and your hands should come to rest just above or behind your buttocks.

8. Gently pull your arms back and down, away from your body while inhaling. This will arch your back slightly backward. You should feel stretching in the arms, shoulders, and chest, and a squeezing sensation in the midback.

9. Exhale and come back to a relaxed position, with your hands still together.

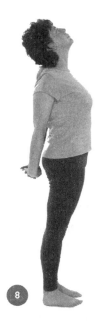

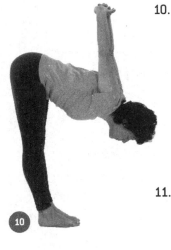

10. Inhale, and then while exhaling, bend forward from the hips, bringing your arms up toward your head as if attempting to stretch your arms all the way over your head while your hands are still interlocked. The bend at the waist should be to the point of feeling stretching in the back of your thighs. Tuck your head slightly and keep the rest of your back straight.

11. Pull your arms up and forward until you feel them stretching. Hold this pose for two to four breaths. With each exhale, gently pull the arms forward toward your head; with each inhale, let the arms relax while you always maintain some forward tension on the arms.

12. Inhale as you come back to a standing position, then exhale as you release your hands and come back into Mountain Pose.

NECK STRETCHING AND RANGE-OF-MOTION EXERCISE

If you have neck problems, this exercise can be very helpful, but it can also cause neck problems to flare up if not done carefully and consciously. If you have neck problems, please consult with your chiropractor before attempting this posture.

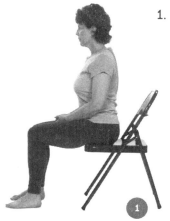

1. You are going to move from the standing position of the previous exercises to a sitting position. Choose a firm chair with a flat surface. Don't lean back onto the backrest; sit on the front one-third of the chair so that you're sitting on your "sitting bones," not your sacrum or tailbone. Your feet should rest flat on the floor, your calves should be perpendicular to the floor, and your thighs should be parallel to the floor. Sit with your back straight, low back pulled forward, chest lifted, shoulders back and relaxed, and head level.

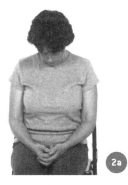

2. Inhale slowly, and while exhaling, let your head bend slowly forward, bringing your chin toward your chest. As you inhale, bring your head back to level. Do this movement one to three times before moving on to the next in the series. With each stretch bring the neck to tension. Don't force the stretch or movement, and don't try to make the joints pop.

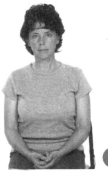

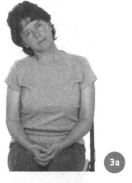

3. While exhaling, slowly bring the right ear toward the right shoulder. Don't raise the shoulder; just allow the head to bend gently sideways. Bring the head back to level while inhaling and then bring the left ear toward the left shoulder. Make sure to stretch both the left and right sides on each repetition. Repeat the same number of times as you did in step 1. Bring the head back to level on the inhale.

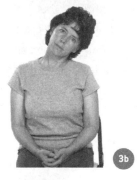

4. The final motion of this exercise is rotation. As you exhale, rotate the head to the right. Slightly decline the head forward while rotating. (This will cause the nose to point down toward the shoulder, instead of pointing straight out over the shoulder.) Rotate until you bring the neck to tension, and hold until completion of the exhale. As with the other motions, inhale while coming back to neutral position. Repeat to the left.

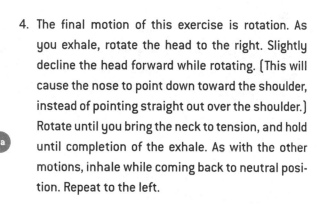

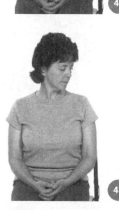

RESTING POSE

Upon completion of your yoga exercises this is one final posture that I strongly recommend. This posture is meant to relax the body and mind. You will need a small hand towel and a blanket for this.

1. Lie on your back with a rolled-up hand towel under your neck to place the neck in a comfortable, slightly extended position. Your arms should rest naturally at your sides, palms facing up. Your legs should be comfortably apart, with your feet and calves relaxed. Place the rolled-up blanket under your knees, raising them about four to six inches off the floor. Don't try to hold your feet pointing up; allow them to relax and point out and away from one another.

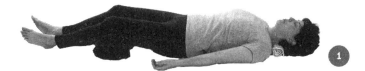

2. Once in this position, make sure you are comfortable and focus on your yoga breath. Relax for three to five minutes.

When yoga is done correctly, its benefits go far beyond just stretching. Much of the benefit gained arises from careful application of the breathing technique associated with each exercise, and with thorough attention to small details. Adding some or all of these exercises not only will support your chiropractic care by strengthening the muscles that surround the spine, but will also improve your flexibility and balance, increase your body's efficiency by providing it with more oxygen, and relax you both mentally and physically.

If you find you enjoy yoga and would like to learn more, there are a wide number of classes, books, videos, and resources available. Today many health clubs (as well as the YMCA and YWCA) offer yoga as an exercise option. However, make sure you check out the class and the teacher. You want someone who can assist you in doing the postures correctly, so there is no danger of overextending your muscles.

Above all, remember that the goal of yoga is a gentle stretch. If you experience any discomfort in any of the postures, ease up. Listen to your body and let it tell you how far it can stretch given its current status. You'll be surprised at how quickly you will be stretching farther and with more ease than you ever thought possible.

▶ Tai Chi and Other Movement Therapies

One of the other forms of exercise that I recommend to my patients because of its benefits for balance, flexibility, and focus is tai chi (pronounced "tie chee"). Over the last forty or so years, tai chi has become a popular movement therapy/exercise in the West. Tai chi has its roots in ancient Chinese culture and is considered one form of an even more ancient practice known as qigong (pronounced "key-gong"). *Qi* refers to life energy, vitality, or life force, and *gong* means to practice, cultivate, or refine, so qigong is the practice of getting in touch with our basic life energy and directing that force to self-healing and enlightenment. The roots of qigong date back to

Chinese prehistory, and many believe that it was originally imported from India. Over many centuries qigong has been adopted and transformed by many religious, spiritual, and academic organizations. Today there are thousands of applications of qigong in the healing, religious, and philosophical traditions of China. Qigong is one of the four pillars of traditional Chinese medicine; the other three are acupuncture, massage, and herbal medicines.

The practice of tai chi that has become well known in the West began as a martial arts practice developed during the seventeenth century in China. Over the past three hundred years it has undergone changes that have removed many of the more forceful elements. Today tai chi consists of 108 separate movements done in a specific order, forming a kind of slow "dance" that is correlated closely with proper breathing technique and precise movement (much like yoga). While there are several kinds of tai chi, most of the variations have created a short form of between twenty and forty movements that a beginner can learn quickly. The short forms are also valuable for older people and those who are ill.

Tai chi has been shown in numerous studies to have a positive effect on lowering blood pressure. Two studies by the National Institute on Aging have shown that older people who practice tai chi have a significantly reduced risk of injury from falling. This was supported by a study from Harvard Medical School that stated tai chi "improve[s] balance, flexibility, muscle strength and reaction time." Additional benefits that have been demonstrated in other studies include stress reduction, better posture, and improved recovery from injuries.

There are many types of tai chi and qigong that you might have access to in your community; tai chi classes are offered at many local colleges, high schools, and YMCAs. Ask your chiropractor to recommend a class, or look in the yellow pages under martial arts.

If yoga and tai chi are not your style, perhaps another form of movement therapy may be more to your liking. Many dance classes can provide the benefits of rhythmic movement, enhanced balance, stress reduction, and so on. For example, square dancing might be one form of exercise that you find enjoyable and beneficial. The most important factor in all exercise is whether or not you enjoy it and will do it on a regular basis. Find something you like doing, and you will continue to do it simply because you enjoy it. Then you'll be far more certain to reap its benefits.

▶ Cardiovascular Health and General Fitness

As you continue to develop your healthy lifestyle, keep remembering the concept of baby steps. If you start out with a fifteen- to thirty-minute yoga routine and then add a cardiovascular routine that lasts another thirty minutes, you are looking at an exercise schedule that will take about one hour three to five days per week. Even though I live a very busy life, I feel this investment of time for my health is reasonable. But *you* are going to have to choose your level of commitment. Understand that the best approach for you is the one *you* will succeed at, one baby step at a time.

When most people think of exercise, they envision two things: cardiovascular or aerobic exercises, and some kind of weight-based, anaerobic strength training. Cardiovascular exercise benefits the health of the heart, lungs, and circulation. It has been proven to reduce the incidence of heart disease, high blood pressure, stroke, obesity, diabetes, and colon cancer. When done correctly, cardiovascular exercise can benefit the joints, muscles, and bones. Aerobic or cardiovascular exercise is also the foundation of almost every sensible weight-loss program. To lose weight, we have to burn more calories than we eat, and aerobic exercise causes us to expend energy at much higher levels. It also can increase our metabolism, so we burn calories faster and more efficiently. Simply adding an aerobic or cardiovascular component to your exercise routine two or three times a week will increase your overall health dramatically.

On the other hand, strength training, or anaerobic exercise, is important for maintaining or increasing bone density, and helps you retain the calcium in your bones. The body is always breaking down and building up bone simultaneously; by putting controlled yet regular stress on the bones, strength training activates the cells that build bones, causing them to become stronger and more organized. Anaerobic exercise has a similar effect on the muscles, creating new fibers while building up the ones that are already there. With strength training, the maximum benefits again require a commitment of two or three sessions a week. These sessions don't have to be prolonged, nor do they have to be so strenuous that you can't walk or lift things afterward. But you do need to make a commitment to regular strength training.

Most programs designed to improve physical fitness consist of three components, represented by the acronym FIT:

- Frequency—how often you exercise
- Intensity—how hard you push yourself
- Time—how long you spend doing it

When it comes to cardiovascular exercise, the American Heart Association (AHA) recommends the following:

- Frequency: three to four times per week
- Intensity: vigorous activity, at 50 to 75 percent of your maximum heart rate
- Time: thirty minutes each session

Remember the spirit of baby steps: Give yourself permission to start small and build up your exercise routine. You might want to begin with just five to ten minutes of cardiovascular exercise and work up to the thirty-minute level. And if you have a personal or family history of cardiovascular problems, always make sure you consult your primary health care provider before engaging in a vigorous exercise program.

When you're choosing the type of cardiovascular activity you wish to undertake on a regular basis, take the health of your spine and joints into consideration, too. Some activities, such as jogging or running on hard surfaces, can be very stressful on the spine and joints, so I recommend that my patients explore the wide range of aerobic choices available. Some suggested types of activity that would be conducive to good spinal health are:

- Brisk walking
- Hiking
- Stair climbing
- Low-impact aerobics
- Bicycling

- Rowing
- Swimming
- Cross-country skiing
- Skiing machines

Other activities and sports that develop good cardiovascular health but are more high-impact are listed below. If you have a history of back problems, it would be best to consult your chiropractor before participating in these activities.

- Running
- Jogging
- Basketball

- Soccer
- Martial arts
- Gymnastics

Common sense can go a long way in determining if a certain form of exercise or activity appears to be overly strenuous on the spine and structure of the body. As we discussed in the yoga section, be aware of your body and how it is responding to a particular form of exercise. There are literally a hundred different kinds of exercise that will promote your cardiovascular health—use your imagination! If you feel your current choice could be harmful, do something else.

For those individuals who cannot exercise vigorously or are currently living a sedentary lifestyle, research has shown that even a moderate or low-intensity increase in activity can have a positive effect on cardiovascular health and lower the risk of heart disease. Here are a few activities that might be your first baby steps in the direction of greater health and fitness.

- Do housework instead of hiring someone
- Work in the yard, or do gardening

- Take a short walk before or after a meal (or both!)
- Stand up while talking on the telephone
- Pedal a stationary bike while watching TV
- Park farther away from the store while shopping
- Take stairs instead of an elevator
- When golfing, walk instead of riding a cart
- Go dancing

I am an enthusiastic fan of walking. If you don't engage in any exercise other than walking (along with some minimal stretching), the health benefits would be substantial. I love to walk. It is good for the heart, lungs, circulation, digestion, joint mobility, strength, and mental health.

If you are just beginning a walking program, I recommend you start with fifteen minutes. The first five minutes should be fairly slow, to warm you up. The middle five minutes should be brisk enough that you feel a slight increase in your heart rate and breathing. The final five minutes is a cool-down period, so walk slower and allow your breathing and heart rate to return to normal. Try to maintain a three-walks-per-week program. Each week, increase the brisk part of the walk by three to five minutes until you reach a total of a forty-minute walk. My wife and I try to complete an hourlong walk three times per week. While we no longer follow this exact prescription of timing, our walks keep us in our target heart range because our route takes us up and down several hills. The scenery is beautiful, and we enjoy each other's company. It makes exercising almost painless! If you are not already walking, I hope that you, too, can start enjoying its many benefits soon.

One of the best things about chiropractic care is that it allows people who have been unable to exercise because of pain to start or resume exercise programs. Rhoda came to my clinic with a history of severe migraines and lower back pain. She also had a weight problem because she couldn't exercise without experiencing extreme discomfort. Within the first few weeks of starting chiropractic care she had 75 percent more movement without pain, and her headaches had gone from four or five a week to one or two every other week. She was able to resume exercising, and she lost 90 pounds over the course of two years. After four years of regular chiropractic care her migraines have disappeared and, she reports, she has "more energy to live a fuller life." I have no doubt that Rhoda's increased energy and well-being can be attributed both to chiropractic care and to her commitment to regular exercise.

▶ Putting Together Your Personal "Baby Steps" Program

Some of my toughest yet most rewarding patients are those who come in and say, "Dr. Lenarz, I know I should exercise and eat well and get regular chiropractic care. But part of me thinks, what's the point? I could get hit by a truck tomorrow. I just want to enjoy life, and all of this seems like a lot of effort."

I tell such patients, "You're right. We all have to go someday, no matter how healthy we are. And taking care of your health does take effort. But if you look at the odds, a healthy lifestyle significantly increases the possibility of a longer life, and certainly a more enjoyable time while we're here. All I can tell you is this: If you *don't* make the effort to be healthy, you increase your chances of feeling lousy and having a shortened life. By choosing consistently to make efforts toward health, you'll increase your chances of living longer and feeling good. For me the choice is easy. What choice will you make?"

Lifestyle changes are not a game; they are about creating a life you are going to enjoy enough to live every day. That's why I believe in the concept of baby steps, making small changes that are easily incorporated in your current lifestyle. Add a little yoga to your morning or evening routine. Take a quick walk at lunchtime or after dinner. Find a sport you enjoy, or someone to exercise with. If you need a little extra support because you have health problems (sore back, cardiovascular issues, and so on), consult your chiropractor and/or primary-care physician and ask them to help you devise an exercise program suited to your particular needs. Follow the guidelines in this chapter, and build your exercise lifestyle change as quickly as is appropriate for you.

The main thing is to get started *now* doing something that you enjoy and can commit to continuing on a regular basis. Once you get into the habit of incorporating exercise into your day, I guarantee that most of the time you'll enjoy it immensely. And when you get the "I don't want to exercise" blues, force of habit will often carry you outside and onto the road, or into the gym—and then you might actually find yourself enjoying exercise in spite of yourself.

9

Eating for a Healthier Life

Every time we turn around it seems we're getting new and often conflicting advice on what to eat, how much to eat, and when and where to eat it. Some of this conflict is due to an explosion of research into nutrition, but another part is due to a lack of agreement among the people and agencies that set nutrition guidelines. Even now, you may hear completely different dietary recommendations from a hospital dietitian, a degreed nutritionist, a naturopath, an OMD (doctor of Oriental medicine), and a chiropractor. The good news is that we are more aware of the effect of nutrition on our overall health; the bad news is that it's difficult to be certain about the nutrition advice we're getting.

I often have seen the impact of this confusion about diet and nutrition on my patients. They come into my office with a clipping from the newspaper on the latest supplement or diet fad and ask, "Do you think this will help my arthritis?" "Will this relieve my pain?" "Could this really help me lose weight?"

Nutrition can play a vital role in the health of our spine and nerves as well as our overall well-being. Although many chiropractors offer nutritional counseling through their offices, I often recommend that my patients consult nutritionists or naturopaths to make changes in their diet and nutrition.

I've also benefited from having a nutrition expert in my family—my wife, Susan. Susan is a registered dietitian, and she has kept up with the latest information and trends in nutritional science. We've often shaken our heads at some of the food fads that people have followed in their quest for health and, often, thinness. But in the same way that chiropractic philosophy endeavors to restore common sense to the field of health care, Susan and I share a desire to bring common sense to the area of nutritional support. We'd like to suggest that you adopt three fundamental understandings when it comes to deciding how to eat.

- **Nutrition doesn't have to be complicated.**   You don't have to know how each vitamin, mineral, and supplement interacts with the body, nor do you have to fulfill every single nutritional requirement at each meal. It's important that you give your body the nutrients it needs, but that doesn't mean you have to adhere to a strict diet or supplement regimen every single day. Understand the importance of nutrition; don't make it an obsession.

- **Use common sense and moderation when it comes to food and nutritional choices.**   Fad diets may be great in the short term, but they usually don't constitute eating plans that will work for the long term. The healthiest people who come into my office are those who eat, exercise, work, and play in moderation. Sure, they can overindulge every so often, but they know the meaning of the "middle way," as the Buddha called it. They listen to their bodies, and follow a few simple principles of choosing foods wisely.

- **Everyone's different.** The plan that works for your friend might not work for you, and the diet you ate in college definitely won't work for you in middle age. Your nutritional choices should be based on your current circumstances. Don't be married to one way of eating. Choose what will work for your current lifestyle. If you consult a nutrition professional, don't be afraid to ask questions or tell the nutritionist your own particular circumstances. That's the only way to get a plan that's right for you.

In this chapter Susan and I want to help you make sense of nutrition in three specific areas. First, we want to talk about how you can use food to support your health. Second, we'll go over some of the major categories of diet plans and discuss their advantages and disadvantages. Third, we'll cover supplements, focusing mainly on those nutrients that can aid in the health of joints, ligaments, tendons, cartilage, muscles, and nerves.

▶ Innate Intelligence and Nutrition

As I pointed out in Chapter 3, our body transforms every food we eat into both the fuel we need to live and the tissues of our body. It uses or converts the right amounts of all nutrients to maintain health and then either stores or excretes the excess. All the nutrients we take in through our food are used to keep our body in balance.

Innate Intelligence, primarily operating through the nervous system, is the master of this internal balance, or *homeostasis.* There are literally thousands of chemical processes going on inside any given cell every second with the sole purpose of maintaining homeostasis. If we go out of balance—because of insufficient nutrition, lack of exercise or rest, subluxation, or a number of other causes—the body does its best to compensate. This compensation, however, can produce a wide range of symptoms. Symptoms are what we experience when the body is attempting to restore itself to homeostasis.

Chiropractic care aligns with the body's desire to restore and maintain homeostasis. Remember that chiropractic's goal is to restore optimal functioning to the body by allowing Innate Intelligence to flow unimpeded by subluxations. But homeostasis also depends on the body receiving the support it needs—good nutrition, adequate water, sleep, exercise, and so on. When we take care of our bodies, we are aligning ourselves with Innate Intelligence.

Just as subluxation can result in disease, so too can significant nutritional imbalances. Many diseases have nutritional components as contributing factors. Yes, we may have genetic predispositions to diabetes, heart disease, and cancer, but study after study shows that we can diminish or worsen our genetic tendencies by our lifestyle choices. Recognizing that our ability to survive is determined by the choices we make gives us power. What we eat and how we act will create either health or disease. When we make a conscious choice to feed our cells instead of our cravings, then we are working in harmony with nature and with the greater design of life.

Many of my patients have used dietary changes to help heal different conditions. For instance, Luella had been under chiropractic care for a long time, using it as one of her primary means of health maintenance. But she was suffering from gallbladder problems and high blood pressure, health concerns that were helped but not eliminated by her chiropractic care. Luella wasn't comfortable with the options provided by conventional medicine—drugs for the blood pressure, surgery for the gallbladder—and went on a quest for alternative means of managing her condition. Her search led her to a doctor of Chinese medicine. He made several dietary recommendations that, quite honestly, didn't make much sense to

Luella: things like avoiding soy, drinking more milk, and eliminat-ing several other foods that seemed unrelated to her symptoms. But sure enough, within a short period of time Luella's blood pres-sure dropped and her gallbladder symptoms disappeared. For the first time she was able to keep her blood pressure down without using medication.

Another patient, Amarah, had been under care for some time for a chronic inflammatory condition that was being managed by chiropractic. Then she was in a car accident. Although we treated her for the effects of the accident, the trauma caused her chronic inflammatory condition to flare up again. Despite our efforts, the condition continued to cause Amarah a lot of pain. She decided to explore other avenues of healing and consulted a nutritionist who was also a medical intuitive. The woman recommended that Ama-rah eliminate all foods of the nightshade family (eggplant, peppers, and tomatoes, for example) from her diet. Within two weeks of changing her diet, Amarah's pain was reduced by 75 percent.

I tell you Luella's and Amarah's stories not to suggest you try their diets but to impress upon you that many conditions have a nutritional component. If you are experiencing anything less than optimal health, you may wish to take a close look at your diet and see if there are changes that need to be made. When we regard food and nutrition as fuel for the body as well as entertainment for the taste buds, then we can make the choices that will lead us to greater health and vitality.

▶Water: The First Nutrient

When thinking about nutrition, most people don't put water at the top of the list, yet we can live a lot longer without food than we can without water. As you probably learned in grade school, the adult human body is about 70 percent water. We need water to maintain homeostasis. If we lose only a small percentage of our body's water, we're in deep trouble. Water is the body's primary solvent and medium of transport. It helps to regulate cell volume, nutrient flow to cells, and removal of wastes. Water is an integral part of the body's temperature regulation mechanism; we also use water in digestion, absorption, and circulation. To stay healthy and move fluidly, our bones and joints must have adequate amounts of water-based fluid surrounding them. Even our nerves communicate by sending signals through a sea of enzymes composed mostly of—you guessed it—water.

Unlike the proverbial camel, however, human beings can't store water for future needs. And since we excrete water when we sweat, urinate, defecate, and with every breath we take, a lot of water (on average, about 10 cups) leaves the body in the course of a given day. To keep ourselves hydrated, we must replace the water we lose. We can do so in several ways. First, almost every single nutritional guide recommends drinking several glasses of water throughout the day. That's water, not beverages such as juice, carbonated beverages, and caffeinated drinks like coffee and tea. These drinks are not processed by the body in the same way that straight water is. If you drink them instead of water you are doing your body a disservice. (In fact, because some soda pop, coffee, and tea may even have a slight diuretic effect and pull water out of the body, they can cancel out any hydrating benefits these beverages may have.) To give your body one of its most important nutritional supports make sure you are drinking plenty of water, at least eight to ten 8-ounce glasses throughout the day. Don't substitute other beverages. If you want to drink soda, tea, coffee, juices, fine; just drink them in addition to water.

We also can add water to our diet by increasing the amount of high-water-content foods we consume. Most fresh fruits and vegetables contain a great deal of water. That's one of the reasons that a food plan rich in fresh fruits and vegetables keeps our digestive and climinative systems in tune—the water and fiber keep things moving, so to speak, and provide plenty of fluid for the stomach and intestines. However, any water you take in by eating high-water-content foods should be in addition to the plain, pure water you are drinking every day.

Here are four quick hints for getting the proper amount of water in your system.

- Don't let thirst be your guide. If you are at all dehydrated (as most of us are), thirst is not a reliable indicator of the need for water. I fill a bottle with my daily water quota and put it within easy reach through the day. It's a simple way to gauge how much water I'm drinking.

- Be certain of the quality of the water you're drinking. Unfortunately, tap water in many communities can also have chemicals or bacteria in it. Well water is often not much better, because the water table in the United States has become contaminated by commercial fertilizers, industrial runoff, and other pollutants. There are several very good water filters available for your home, or you can choose to buy bottled water. The few pennies these precautions cost are more than worth it when you consider how much of your body is composed of the water you drink.

- One way to tell if you are getting enough water is to check the color of your urine—it should be almost clear. When you first increase your water intake, you may feel like you have to run to the bathroom every hour. That's a normal response; it will take the body a little time to get accustomed to the increased amount of water.

- Depending on your circumstances, you may need *more* water than eight to ten glasses a day. If you exercise vigorously, or live in a warm or extremely dry climate, you will be excreting more water and thus need to drink more to replace it. If you are ill, often one of the most effective aids to recovery is simply to keep yourself well hydrated. I have some patients who, whenever they experience any kind of pain or discomfort, will immediately drink several glasses of water to see if dehydration is contributing to their condition.

Dehydration also can cause a wide range of symptoms that don't seem directly connected to a lack of water. Heart and circulatory difficulties, digestive problems, constipation, even some respiratory symptoms may have inadequate hydration as a contributing cause. And since our eliminatory systems—the ones that flush toxins out of the body—depend on water to function efficiently, insufficient water can put additional strain on the kidneys and liver.

Oxygen is the first requirement the body needs to live, but water is the second. The best thing you can do to support your life, your health, and your chiropractic care is to drink enough water every day.

▶ Food: The Drug You Take Every Day

Food is the primary source of the forty-five to fifty nutrients the body needs to function properly. Unfortunately, what we choose to put in our mouths is not necessarily chosen with its survival value in mind.

I call food "the drug you take every day" for several reasons. First, the nutrients in food—or the lack of them—can affect the body's health and well-being far more than most of the drugs prescribed by conventional medical practitioners. For example, if a pregnant woman doesn't get enough folic acid (a B vitamin), her child is at greater risk for a serious birth defect called neural tube disorder. On the other hand, too much sodium (another mineral essential for the body) can make you retain water and create a system imbalance that can damage the heart muscle.

But food is a drug in other ways as well. Just like recreational drugs, people take food because of the way it makes them feel. Most people choose food based not on nutritive value but on other factors, such as craving and convenience. If this weren't true, then the fast-food and snack industries wouldn't be the billion-dollar businesses they are—and most citizens of the United States wouldn't be fighting obesity, heart disease, diabetes, cancer, and many other diseases that are at least partly caused by the long-term effects of lousy nutrition.

But, as I said earlier, proper nutrition does not have to be complicated. To support your body, begin by recalling the seven "building blocks" your body needs to create all of the substances it needs to function.

- **Carbohydrates.**   Carbohydrates are the body's primary fuel. All carbohydrates are composed of different combinations of sugar molecules, which are converted into glucose (another form of sugar) by the body for use as energy. Carbs come in three forms: simple, complex, and dietary fiber. This classification is based on the number of sugar units contained in each carbohydrate molecule and how the sugars are linked.

  Simple carbohydrates have only one or two units of sugar per molecule. Simple carbs include fructose (the sugar in most fruits), lactose (produced when we digest milk), and disaccharides (found in sugar, honey, and most sweeteners). Sugar molecules in simple carbohydrates are converted almost immediately by the body into glucose.

  Complex carbohydrates have more than two units of sugar per molecule. It takes longer for the body to break apart complex carbohydrate molecules and transform them into glucose; therefore, complex carbs are a steadier energy source than simple carbs. Complex carbs include raffinose and stachyose (sugars found in potatoes, beans, and beets), and starch (found in potatoes, pasta, grains, and rice). Unprocessed sources of complex carbohydrates—whole grains, brown rice, and oatmeal, for example—take longer for the body to process than refined versions of the same foods, and also provide more naturally occurring vitamins and minerals.

  Dietary fiber also has more than two units of sugar per molecule, but the sugars are linked in such a way that they cannot be broken down in the digestive tract, so fiber provides little to no fuel for the body. Fiber is essential for the health of the digestive system. Eaten in proper quantities, fiber helps to slow down the rate of release of nutrients during digestion, allowing the body more time to absorb the nutritional components. Fiber also helps in the elimination of toxins from the digestive tract, "sweeping" the small intestine and colon clean.

- **Protein.**   Protein is used by the body to build, repair, and replace tissue. Every cell in the body contains protein; such vital substances as enzymes, hemoglobin, collagen, and certain hormones are almost entirely protein. Protein is composed of amino acids, and the human body needs about twenty different kinds of amino acids to live. Nine of the essential amino acids cannot be produced in the body and must be obtained from food. While most Americans think of meat and dairy products as our primary sources of protein, most of the world's population get their protein from sources such as legumes, grains, and soybean products like tofu.

- **Fats.**   Fats are the most concentrated source of calories that we consume. Dietary fat (which comes in two main forms, saturated and unsaturated) is converted by the body into essential fatty acids that help control blood pressure, blood clotting, and inflammation. Fat is necessary in cell walls and in the production of hormones. It is also the way the body stores energy for use in the future, and it helps insulate the body from temperature changes. We need a certain amount of fat in our diet to transport and utilize vitamins A, D, and E. However, the amounts and kinds of fats we eat can have a substantial impact on our overall health. As we'll discuss later, most Americans consume a diet that is far too high in saturated and/or hydrogenated fats, which are found in many processed foods. This dietary imbalance has contributed to the current epidemic of obesity and heart-related health problems.

- **Vitamins and minerals.**   These substances allow each and every bodily activity, from movement to structural construction to metabolization to communication between cells, to take place. Many of these important substances interact with each other as well—for example, vitamin D helps calcium move from the digestive tract to the bloodstream and into the bones. Vitamins and minerals are found, to some degree, in most of the foods we eat. But many people (including me) believe that because our diets are less than optimal and many of our food sources nutritionally inadequate, we must take supplements to ensure we are getting all the vitamins and minerals we need.

Nowadays naturally occurring substances called *phytochemicals* are the subject of much study in the field of nutrition. Phytochemicals are found in plants and include a wide range of nutrients beneficial to human health. Phytochemicals such as lycopene (found in red peppers and tomatoes), anthocyanin (found in blueberries), chlorophyllin, saponin, antioxidants, and essential fatty acids can help lower cholesterol, reduce cell damage, stimulate the immune system, lower blood pressure, and protect against aging and cancer. While scientists are endeavoring to reproduce a wide variety of phytochemicals in the laboratory, your best sources for these important nutrients are fruits, vegetables, whole grains, and legumes.

• **Water.** We already talked about the importance of drinking enough water, but we also get a percentage of the water the body needs from food.

Our nutritional needs are not constant. Instead, they vary depending upon lifestyle, age, level of activity, gender, sometimes even ethnicity. One thing is constant, however: We all do better when we have the highest-quality nutrition possible to support ourselves physically. There are a few simple principles that can guide your choices in this area.

• **A good diet is a balanced diet.** If you're not getting all seven nutritional substances—carbs, protein, fats, vitamins, minerals, water, and fiber—in healthful proportions, there's going to be trouble. The best way to ensure you are getting what your body needs is to choose a wide variety of foods from each category.

- **Unprocessed, whole foods are usually better for you than processed foods.** Too much of the food we eat has been processed to the point of having next to no nutritional value. Plus, many times processing also eliminates other important components of a healthy diet, such as water and fiber, and adds components we don't need, like excess sugar and salt. Take the difference between instant mashed potatoes and a baked potato. The instant potatoes have almost no fiber, lots of salt and sugar, and a whole series of additives such as artificial flavorings. The baked potato, on the other hand, has a moderate number of calories, no added salt or sugar (unless you add it yourself), and more fiber (especially if you eat the skin). The more you buy in the produce section and the less you buy in the processed food sections, the healthier your diet will be.

- **Consider the source of your food.** In this era of agribusiness and factory farms, our fruits and vegetables are often grown in nutrient-poor soil, saturated with petrochemical fertilizers and insecticides, and picked long before they're ripe simply because they'll ship better that way. The animals and fish we eat are stuffed full of hormones and chemicals we would never allow ourselves or our children to take, yet we eat these substances in our meat without a thought.

In the same way that I advocate drinking clean, purified water, I would recommend that you buy organic produce wherever possible. Organic produce is raised in fields where no chemical fertilizers have been used for three years or more. Only natural means of fertilization and pest control are allowed. Organic produce may be a little more expensive, and you may not be able to get every kind of fruit or vegetable throughout the year. But you can consume your produce knowing that you are getting good nutrition without a petrochemical soup to go along with it.

Many of the same stores that sell organic produce also carry hormone-free meat, free-range poultry, and non-farm-raised fish. The good news about both organic produce and "clean" meats and seafood is that they have more and better flavor than their factory-farmed counterparts. If you really want to enjoy your food while you get the best nutrition from the cleanest source, try organic.

- **Eat on a regular schedule whenever possible, and allow yourself time to eat.**   There have been dozens of studies describing the effects of our modern hurry-up lifestyle on our ability to absorb and enjoy our food. Our bodies spend an amazing amount of energy to process the food we eat; in fact, digestion consumes more energy than almost any other biological process. To get the most from our food, we need to support our bodies in two ways. First, eating small, regular meals throughout the day is easier on the body than the typical American schedule of skipping breakfast, racing through lunch, then eating a big dinner right before we go to bed. (In fact, if you want to lose weight, it's actually better to eat your larger meals earlier in the day and eat nothing completely after 8 P.M.) A schedule of small, regular meals puts less strain on the digestive system.

Second, take time to eat and enjoy your food. A great deal of digestion is done in the mouth, as the teeth break the food down mechanically and the enzymes in saliva do the same thing chemically. Chewing your food thoroughly and letting your body have time to digest what you're eating supports your digestive system. Rushing through a meal, shoving food in your mouth, chewing it just enough so you can swallow it, then bolting from the table the minute you're done is a recipe for inadequate digestion and absorption. It can also produce conditions such as chronic indigestion, gas, bloating, constipation, and so on. (By the way, it takes approximately twenty minutes for the stomach to recognize that it's full and signal the brain to tell you to stop eating. Therefore, taking longer to eat a meal means less risk of overeating when you've already had enough.)

• **Eat to live, don't live to eat.**   Believe me, I enjoy eating as much as the next person, but I also believe that food is designed mainly to nourish my body. When you choose what to eat simply based on whatever you're craving and you don't take nutrition into account, you can quickly find yourself in deep trouble—overweight, undernourished, with all kinds of physical problems. Nutrition isn't rocket science; it's easy to create a balanced diet that is also satisfying. But you've got to make feeding your body the priority, not satisfying your tastebuds' every whim.

▶ Which Eating Plan Is Right for You?

Every year it seems there is a new diet plan being promoted by some expert or other who tells us that everything we thought we knew about the optimal diet is wrong and that he or she has the key to thinness, health, and vitality. On the other hand, we have the government's food pyramid and RDA (recommended daily allowance) for the amount of vitamins and minerals we need— recommendations that change with glacierlike slowness and only after massive amounts of pressure by nutritionists and dieticians.

What are we to do? Should we try the "meat, no potatoes" plan for a while, then switch to the "potatoes, no meat" version? Should we gulp down multiple vitamins and minerals, adding a few extra herbal supplements just to make sure we're getting enough nutritional support no matter how lousy our diet may be? Should we do without a meal, or eat every two hours? Should we take a scientific approach and calculate every calorie as well as every microgram of vitamins C, D, E, B$_{12}$, and so on or say the heck with it and eat what we darn well please?

I'd like to advocate a little common sense when it comes to choosing your eating plan. In this section we're going to look at some of the basic trends in nutrition and discuss the pros and cons of each. We'll go over the USDA food pyramid recommendations. We'll discuss eating plans that emphasize protein (Atkins), those that advocate high-carbohydrate/low-fat consumption (Ornish), and diets that focus on specific proportions of protein to carbohydrate to fat (the Zone). We'll investigate vegetarian diets and their effect on the body. I hope that by the end of our discussion you'll have enough high-quality information to choose an eating plan based upon your individual circumstances and needs.

The USDA Food Pyramid

In 1992 the U.S. Department of Agriculture (USDA) changed its nutritional recommendations for the first time in over sixty years. It created what's now called the food pyramid, which serves as the suggested guide for a healthy diet for all Americans. The food pyramid divides foods into six basic groups and suggests the relative amounts of each we should consume each day (see page 174).

While the basics of the food pyramid are widely accepted because they seem to suggest a varied diet and plenty of fruits and vegetables, a number of respected nutritionists and dieticians take issue with its recommendations. The problem with the food pyramid, they say, is a lack of specificity in both the different categories of food and the quality of foods in each area. For instance, there is little to no emphasis placed on choosing complex carbohydrates such as whole-grain breads and pastas, brown rice, and so on, over simple carbohydrates found in breads and pastas made from processed white flour. Potatoes are considered a vegetable in the food pyramid, where in many cases they should more appropriately be called a starch.

Other nutritionists take issue with the lack of emphasis on choosing low-fat dairy products and lean meats. They point to the alarming incidence of high cholesterol in many segments of the U.S. population and say that advocating unsaturated rather than saturated fats could go a long way to making Americans healthier

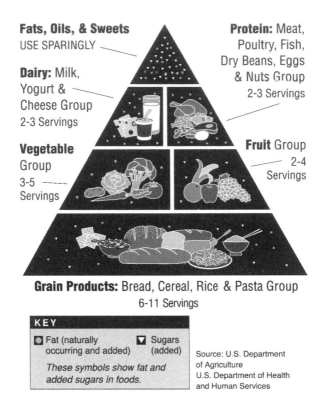

Fats, Oils, & Sweets
USE SPARINGLY

Dairy: Milk, Yogurt & Cheese Group
2-3 Servings

Vegetable Group
3-5 Servings

Protein: Meat, Poultry, Fish, Dry Beans, Eggs & Nuts Group
2-3 Servings

Fruit Group
2-4 Servings

Grain Products: Bread, Cereal, Rice & Pasta Group
6-11 Servings

KEY

☐ Fat (naturally occurring and added)   ▼ Sugars (added)

These symbols show fat and added sugars in foods.

Source: U.S. Department of Agriculture
U.S. Department of Health and Human Services

in general. To top it all off, a growing body of research suggests that whether the food pyramid is good or bad, Americans aren't following it anyway. Most of us get anywhere from 27 to 45 percent of our calories from the high-fat, sugary foods at the top of the pyramid, and up to 97 percent of us don't get the recommended number of servings of fruits and vegetables on any given day.

The food pyramid does advocate a varied and balanced way of eating, but I would like to suggest that you consider the sources of the food choices you make, and go for the highest quality. Whole grains are better than refined, processed ones. Unsaturated fats such as olive oil are better than butter or margarine (especially since margarine contains trans fatty acids, substances that are very harmful to your circulatory system). Low-fat protein and dairy sources provide more nutritional value per ounce than high-fat choices. And the wider the variety of fruits and vegetables you eat—making sure to include dark green vegetables as well as yellow and orange fruits and vegetables—the more nutrients per calorie you will consume.

High-Carbohydrate/
Low-Fat Eating Plans

Dean Ornish is probably the best-known advocate for a diet regimen that has been very popular for the last twenty-five years. This plan recommends eating primarily vegetables, grains, and other complex carbohydrates, and using fats and animal protein sparingly. This low-animal-fat diet has been proven over time to decrease cholesterol levels in those who have had problems with cholesterol in the past. The Ornish approach is reflected somewhat in the USDA food pyramid. The Pritikin diet (which is extremely low in fat) is another example of this kind of eating plan.

If you look at cultures around the world, most of them eat in just this way. In societies across Asia and Africa, most people eat a diet based primarily on complex carbohydrates such as unrefined grains, accompanied by a fairly wide variety of fruits and vegetables. Fats, animal protein, and dairy products are used for seasoning rather than as the main component of a meal. Refined sugar is used sparingly.

In America, the low-fat/high-complex-carbohydrate approach is given a lot of lip service, but very few people actually follow its recommendations. Yes, we eat a lot of carbohydrates, but most of them are almost completely empty of fiber and any other nutritive value. The typical American diet is composed of fast food, refined sugar in the form of desserts and sodas, and way too much fat. In fact, most of the vegetables consumed in the United States are potatoes—eaten in the form of french fries or potato chips!

The low-fat/high-carbohydrate style of eating may be helpful for anyone who has heart or circulatory problems. However, many people find it difficult to maintain the extremely low levels of fat allowed in this particular diet. Diabetics and other people who have issues with blood sugar may also have problems (see the next section). It's important to note that if you eliminate all animal fats (including dairy products) and vegetable oils, you remove many of the food sources of the fat-soluble vitamins A, D, E, and K.

As with any eating plan, you may need to fine-tune the low-fat/high-carbohydrate approach to suit your own needs. In some specific circumstances, this diet may not provide enough protein or fat. Pregnant or breastfeeding women, for example, may need more protein or fat to keep themselves and their babies nourished. Someone who does a lot of weight lifting or bodybuilding also may need more protein.

If you do choose to adopt this diet, emphasize fruits and vegetables, and make sure that the grains you eat are mostly whole grains such as whole wheat, brown rice, or oatmeal rather than processed products like white bread, pasta, and white rice. Not only will you get a significant nutritional boost from the vitamins and minerals in the grains, but the fiber they contain will help even out the rate of absorption of food in the body, keeping blood sugar levels on an even keel. It also might be smart to add a general vitamin and mineral supplement to your regimen. However, a diet rich in complex, unrefined carbohydrates such as grains, vegetables, and whole fruits, spiced up with judicious amounts of unsaturated fats and proteins, in general is a sensible approach to healthy eating.

The Zone: 30/30/40 Eating

There has been a great deal of dissatisfaction in parts of the nutrition community with the high-carbohydrate approach to eating. "Americans have known about low-fat, high-carbohydrate diets for years, and we're still getting fatter," they say. "Something's wrong. Either we can't follow the diet because it's too strict, or the diet itself is affecting the body in a negative way." One of the problems that have been associated with a high-carbohydrate diet is that it has a tendency to increase the body's production and storage of fat.

Food is either converted to energy, used to build tissue, or stored as fat. When you eat carbohydrates, they are converted to glucose (sugar) by the digestive process, and then transported throughout the body by the bloodstream. Glucose is the body's source of instant energy. An increase of glucose in the blood signals the pancreas to secrete insulin.

Insulin has two primary roles. First, it helps glucose get into almost every cell in the body. Second, insulin signals the liver when too much glucose has entered the system. In response, the liver converts the extra glucose into another chemical called glycogen, which is stored in the liver and muscles. Glycogen turns back into glucose as needed to provide fuel for the body between meals. But the body can only use so much glucose at one time, and can only store so much glycogen before it gets overloaded. When that happens, the liver converts any extra glucose into fat.

Some nutritionists feel that eating too many carbohydrates, especially refined sugars and starchy grains and vegetables, can cause insulin levels to become consistently elevated. They theorize that this can produce what's called *insulin resistance syndrome.* The body becomes desensitized to high levels of insulin, resulting in glucose being converted more readily into fat instead of being stored as glycogen or used as energy. These same nutritionists feel that there is a better way to balance the diet and avoid the overproduction of insulin and fat.

Proteins and fats do not have the same effect as carbohydrates. They do not raise blood sugar levels as dramatically and do not trigger the release of large quantities of insulin. Therefore, the theory goes, if you eat proteins, fats, and carbohydrates in specific ratios, your blood sugar will remain within a healthy range and your insulin levels will remain relatively constant. This will allow you to use the nutrients in your food in the most effective way and keep your liver from converting so many calories into fat for storage.

That's the premise behind Barry Sears' Zone 30/30/40 diet. Sears recommends that each meal contain 30 percent low-fat protein, 30 percent fat (mostly unsaturated), and 40 percent carbohydrates (in the form of fruits and nonstarchy vegetables). He also limits the amount of grain-based carbohydrates such as breads, pastas, rice, and other starches. He believes these carbohydrates convert to glucose too quickly and cause an unhealthy rise in blood sugar levels. Finally, Sears discourages consumption of most dairy products because they, too, cause the body to produce glucose quickly. Eggs, egg whites, low-fat cheeses, and milk are allowed in limited quantities.

Millions of people swear by the Zone diet, and it does have its advantages. It's far more balanced and healthy than the current dietary habits of most Americans, because its primary sources of calories are low-fat proteins, healthy sources of unsaturated fats (like olive or canola oil, some nuts, and avocados), and fruits and vegetables. Its schedule of three meals a day plus snacks means that your blood sugar level will probably stay fairly level, preventing the highs and lows many people experience when they eat too many carbohydrates. And certainly, if you wish to lose weight, filling up on low-fat protein and fruits and vegetables usually works wonders. However, if your health problems tend more toward high cholesterol than blood sugar irregularities, levels of dietary fat at 30 percent may be a little high (although the current American average is 27 to 45 percent). If the Zone diet appeals to you, try it. Just make sure you stick to its recommendations for both portion size and food quality (low-fat protein and unsaturated fat), and add a basic vitamin-mineral supplement for insurance.

High-Protein/Low-Carbohydrate Diets

Every so often the world of nutrition seems to return to high-protein diets. The Atkins diet was popular in the 1960s and is now back on the best-seller lists. The so-called Mayo Clinic diet was a fad for a while, and in 2000, the Schwarzbein diet was creating a stir. All of these diets tell us carbs are the enemy, and protein and fat are what our bodies truly need to attain health and slimness. With high-protein eating plans, you are supposed to eat protein at every meal and restrict your carbohydrates significantly. Some high-protein plans suggest you eliminate sugars and starchy carbohydrates completely and get most of your carbohydrates from nonstarchy vegetables and fruits alone.

High-protein diets are supposed to make you healthier in three ways. First, by eliminating most starchy carbohydrates you keep your blood sugar more level. (That's one of the reasons some diabetics follow a high-protein regimen.) Second, when the body doesn't have carbohydrates as a source of instant energy (in the form of glycogen), it starts burning its own fat reserves instead. The result: a slimmer, leaner body. Third, many of the toxins the body takes in through food, water, and air are locked in the fat stores. When these fat stores are burned as energy, the toxins are burned as well.

One of the reasons that high-protein diets have been around for so long is that they help people lose weight fairly quickly. The problem, however, is the *way* in which they cause people to lose weight. High-protein, high-fat diets cause the body to lose stored water. This loss of water is the reason these diets can produce a dramatic drop in weight so quickly. Another problem with this type of diet is that it causes the body to use up its store of glycogen, which leads to the burning of stored fat. Although this may seem like a good thing, it causes some additional problems. When we begin to use up the body's store of fats, it causes an alternation in metabolism called *ketosis.* Ketosis means the overproduction of ketones, or acid-based molecules, which circulate throughout the bloodstream and then are excreted in the urine. Over the short term, ketosis does help you get slimmer. But over the long term, ketosis can cause a systemic poisoning of the body called *ketoacidosis,* with symptoms that include nausea, dehydration, mental confusion, and even coma.

Another problem with high-protein, high-fat diets has to do with the kinds of fats consumed. Many of the protein and fat sources recommended by diets such as Atkins, Mayo, and Schwarzbein are high in saturated fats. Bacon, cheese, most meats, and cream are all on the list as accepted foods, and many of the diets say you can eat fairly large quantities of such items. But, doctors say, this much saturated fat will cause most people's cholesterol levels to shoot through the roof, and high cholesterol has been linked with problems of the heart and circulatory system.

The high-protein, high-fat diet proponents counter that most of our cholesterol is formed within the body, by the liver, and that eating carbohydrates rather than fat actually causes the liver to produce *more* cholesterol, not less. Not eating enough fat in the diet signals the body that this is a time of famine, and to increase its fat reserves just in case. The liver then increases its production of cholesterol. Conversely, eating enough fat as a part of your diet prevents this signal being given. The liver cranks down its production of cholesterol, fewer calories are converted to stored fat, and proper balance is maintained.

Because meats and fats are pretty low in fiber (and, of course, they contain none of the essential phytochemicals present in veggies and fruits), these diets usually include a certain amount of nonstarchy vegetables to be eaten at almost every meal. If you choose to follow one of these plans, make sure you eat all the vegetables recommended. Also, your best guide to eating is your body's response to your diet of choice. Some people love this diet because it makes them feel full. Others can't stomach the amount of concentrated protein and fat at every meal. Keep evaluating your response to the diet, and don't be afraid to change if you feel it is not supporting your health as you would like. Finally, I do recommend that with any extreme change in eating, you check with a nutrition professional. Your chiropractor may provide nutrition counseling, or be able to recommend someone with experience in the eating plan you are following.

Vegetarianism

A lot of different diets fall under the category of vegetarianism. Some people eat no animal products or fish at all. Others eat fish but no meat. Others eat eggs and dairy. Others call themselves vegetarians because they only eat chicken and fish once in a while. All of these eating plans, however, share an emphasis on fruits, vegetables, and grains as the primary sources of nutrition.

A vegetarian way of eating can be very healthy, since we get high quantities of vitamins and minerals from vegetable sources. The major concern for most vegetarians is the quantity and quality of protein in their diet. Protein is present in a wide variety of vegetable sources—soy, beans and legumes, and even some grains (whole wheat provides approximately 5 grams of protein per serving). The proteins in grains and legumes combine to provide the complete range of amino acids required by the body. Vegetable protein sources lack many of the negative aspects of some animal proteins, notably high levels of saturated fat, while offering increased amounts of beneficial phytochemicals. In fact, soy protein can have additional benefits for women because it contains a natural plant form of estrogen, a key hormone before, during, and after menopause.

Vegetarians used to be told that it was important to eat grains and legumes together, in order to get the exact ratio of essential amino acids provided by animal sources. However, recent research indicates that this is not necessarily true. As long as grains and legumes are eaten within a few hours of each other, the body can combine them and produce the essential amino acids as a part of the digestive process. In other words, you could have grains for breakfast and legumes for lunch and still get the right nutrients for amino acid production. Vegetarians who include a modest amount of fish, eggs, or dairy products in their diets are less at risk of protein deficiencies.

It is true that many vegetable sources of protein are not as concentrated as animal sources, because beans, grains, and legumes contain a great deal more fiber. If you choose to eat a strict vegetarian diet, make sure you (1) consume an adequate amount of high-quality vegetable protein each day, and (2) use supplements (especially the B vitamins) to ensure your body has the full range of amino acids it needs.

The suggestions I made at the beginning of this section hold true for vegetarian diets as well. First, make sure your diet contains a wide variety of vegetables, fruits, grains, legumes, fats, and so on. Second, consider the quality of the food you're eating. A fruit bar you buy at the health food store may be completely vegan but still contain high levels of fat and added sugar in the form of fructose, honey, or other simple sugars. It's better to eat whole foods that are processed as little as possible. Third—and this is very important—not everyone is cut out for a vegetarian diet. Some people feel light, healthy, and energetic on this eating plan. Others feel like they have no energy; they're sluggish and their minds are foggy. Still others feel deprived and emotionally strung out. If vegetarianism isn't right for you, don't worry about it. There's no right or wrong in eating—only what's best for your own particular physiology.

A few final words about eating plans: First, no matter what plan you choose, watch your refined sugar intake. All the evidence indicates that refined sugar is a major problem in our society. It is a proven contributing factor to the epidemic incidence of obesity. Refined sugar not only adds empty calories to our diet, but also creates an instant flood of insulin as the body rushes to handle the influx of straight glucose. Sugar actually robs the body of nutrients because it takes so many nutrients to metabolize it. There are no health benefits to eating refined sugar, yet on average Americans consume 149 pounds of it per person per year. If you want to support your health and vitality, one of the best things you can do is to eliminate refined sugar from your diet. And one of the easiest ways to eliminate refined sugar is to cut way down on processed foods. Sodas, fruit-flavored soft drinks, spaghetti sauce, cold cereals, salad dressing, bread products, even processed meats can contain refined sugar in the form of fructose, corn syrup, or glucose. If you choose to eat processed food, learn to be a careful reader of labels so that you know exactly what you're eating.

Second, the human body is immensely adaptable. Our bodies can synthesize energy from almost every kind of food, from the worst junk food to the healthiest meal ever served. We have adapted our diet to our circumstances for millennia. For example, Inuit peoples in the Arctic used to live most of their lives eating fish and whale blubber. Other cultures—some Hindu sects in the southern part of India, for example—eat grains and vegetables almost exclusively, consuming no meat at all. There are at least as many diets as there are peoples and cultures on the earth. So don't feel that you have to eat in a particular way to be healthy. Use balance, variety, and moderation as your watchwords, and you'll probably come up with a way of eating that will work for you.

Third, if you're not happy with the results you're getting with your current eating plan, change it! Sometimes it's good to shake up your system a little; it can help you learn more about your body and what it needs. Remember, your needs may change depending on your circumstances. What you ate as a teenager might cause you to put on a lot of extra weight by the time you're in your thirties or forties. Don't be afraid to do something different if you're not getting the energy you want from what you eat. Do some research, determine your direction and goals, and find an eating plan that supports you. Your body will adapt.

▶ Weight Loss: The Great American Pursuit

As a chiropractor, I've seen the detrimental effects in my patients of being overweight or obese. Not only are there proven cardiovascular, respiratory, and digestive risks to being overweight, but those extra pounds also place increased stress on the entire musculoskeletal system. While obesity may be caused by many factors— among them genetic predisposition, inadequate digestion and/or assimilation, psychological issues, and other factors—there is one cause present in almost every case: *The body is taking in more calories than it is expending.* No matter how much or how little you eat, to lose weight you have to use more energy than is being provided by the food (energy) you are taking in. That's why I advocate regular aerobic and weight-bearing exercise for anyone who wishes to lose weight.

Aerobic exercise literally turns up your metabolism and increases your body's ability to use the fuel you provide it. As I said in Chapter 8, in the first few minutes of aerobic exercise, you are burning carbohydrates—they're like the kindling your body uses to get its fire started. Once the fire is hot enough, the body throws logs, or stored fat, on the fire so it can keep going for a long time. When you combine regular aerobic exercise with strength training (which builds lean muscle mass and strengthens bones), you are helping your body to function at peak efficiency. And unless there is some underlying genetic or physiological imbalance, as long as you continue to use more calories than you take in, the weight will come off.

Exercise takes care of the energy expenditure side of the weight equation. However, most people trying to lose weight can also choose to make some changes in their eating habits, either temporarily or permanently. Indeed, people usually adopt eating plans such as Atkins, Ornish, Schwarzbein, or the Zone with the goal of losing weight. Since we've already discussed the pros and cons of a wide variety of plans, I want to add only a few quick points.

First, whatever eating plan you choose, make sure it provides you with enough nutrients, calories, and water to lose weight gradually and healthfully. So-called crash diets, like three-day juice regimens, the tomatoes/protein/grapefruit diet, or even fasting, can create a quick but ultimately illusory weight loss, often due to loss of water stored in the body. Also, a drastic, sudden reduction in calories puts the body into what's called famine mode. To conserve itself in a perceived famine, the body starts using fewer calories to operate. So when you start eating even a little bit more, all those calories go straight to fat (stored to prevent starvation in the next famine time). Efficient, certainly—but it means that starvation diets can actually make you fatter because you store more of your food as fat reserves. Most experts agree that a weight loss of a pound or two a week is a healthful, attainable goal.

Second, and very important, whatever eating plan you choose, make sure it provides balance, variety, and satisfaction. Otherwise, you won't be able to stick to it for very long, and your "miracle diet" will become just another fad you tried and discarded in the search for thinness.

Third, remember that a healthy weight for you may not be the same as for your co-worker, spouse, friend, sister, or brother. Your optimal weight may be ten or twenty pounds over (or under) the established norms for someone of your height. Additionally, your optimal weight may be more than you'd *like* to weigh, based on what you see in magazines and on television. My job as a chiropractor is to support you in living the healthiest, most vital life possible in a body that is functioning at peak efficiency—the body that is uniquely right for you.

▶ Supplements: Use Your Common Sense

Nowadays even conventional medical doctors are becoming more open to the use of supplements in supporting health. M.D.'s are prescribing vitamins and minerals, even recommending that their patients take herbs and other substances such as garlic pills, gingko biloba, St. John's wort, and saw palmetto. Of course, alternative medical practitioners have been advocating the use of high-quality supplements for years. You need to be aware of the effects of a wide range of vitamins, minerals, and herbs so you can make informed choices about what to take and why.

As a chiropractor (with a dietician for a wife), I am aware of the value of supplements to enhance the elements of health I'm most directly concerned with: nerves, bones, and joints. I also know there is an enormous amount of very confusing information concerning supplements and their proper use. Usually I recommend my patients take a good multivitamin-mineral supplement that provides at least 100 percent of the RDA (recommended daily allowance). However, many of my patients also want specific information on how vitamins and minerals can support their chiropractic care. Therefore I am including a brief overview of some of the most common supplements.

Vitamins

Vitamin C is essential for all body functions. It boosts the body's immune system response, and is especially important in healing injured tissue. It also helps maintain the connective tissue of the body, and therefore it is critical for the health of our bones, joints, and skin. It's also involved in fat metabolism, iron absorption, and converting amino acids to serotonin (one of the "feel-good" neurotransmitters produced in the brain). Vitamin C is recognized as a free-radical scavenger and antioxidant. Most of us know about using megadoses of vitamin C to help fight a cold, but various studies have shown that vitamin C also can help alleviate symptoms associated with arthritis, Parkinson's disease, asthma, and various skin diseases. Too much vitamin C has been linked to diarrhea and, in some cases, the development of kidney stones. However, because the RDA of vitamin C is very low, many people find that additional vitamin C (up to 500 mg) can provide many benefits with little to no downside.

Vitamin D is known as the bone-building vitamin because of its role in boosting calcium and phosphorus absorption (essential for the formation of bone). It's also important in preventing bone loss as we grow older. Vitamin D is actually manufactured inside our bodies, but the process requires exposure to sunlight. If you live in a cloudy climate (as I do) or in a place where winter lasts a long time, if your work requires you to be inside a majority of the time, or if you are dark-skinned, you may need additional vitamin D. Most multivitamin supplements contain vitamin D, and milk and other dairy products often are fortified with vitamin D.

The *B vitamins* are involved in energy metabolism, manufacture of neurotransmitters, and neurological and brain functioning. Vitamin B_6 helps the body use protein to make new cells and has been proven to reduce symptoms in people with carpal tunnel syndrome. In some studies, vitamin B_{12} has been shown to improve visual and auditory responses in multiple sclerosis patients. B_{12} deficiency in the elderly can cause depression and other symptoms that may be mistaken for Alzheimer's disease. Some of the B vitamins (notably B_{12}) are found only in meat, eggs, and dairy products, so it's important for vegans to take B-vitamin supplements.

Vitamin E is another powerful antioxidant, helping the body to protect its cells from free-radical damage. The body does not manufacture vitamin E, so we must consume it in one form or another, either in supplements or through our food. This vitamin has proved helpful to people with arthritis, cataracts, cystic fibrosis, and acne. Most health practitioners believe that supplementing the diet with vitamin E can help improve overall health and resistance to cell damage associated with pollution, aging, and some diseases.

Vitamin K (known as the substance that helps our blood clot) also has a role in maintaining bone density.

Essential Fatty Acids (EFAs)

Essential fatty acids are vital to proper nerve functioning in the body. They help form the myelin sheath, which encloses our nerves and permits swift transmission of impulses from branch nerves to the spinal cord to the brain. Flaxseed oil, borage oil, and evening primrose oil are all high in essential fatty acids. Certain fish, such as salmon, are also high in omega-3 oils, which are needed by the body to produce so-called good (HDL) cholesterol (the kind that protects rather than clogs your arteries).

While Americans are notorious for eating a high-fat diet, the kinds of fats we consume are not the kinds we need. We tend to eat processed foods full of hydrogenated fats, which are some of the worst culprits in clogging our arteries and creating the many conditions associated with high cholesterol. Consuming an adequate amount of EFAs each day will help eliminate some of the detrimental effects of hydrogenated fats and promote greater overall health. I recommend adding a teaspoon or so of flaxseed oil to the diet on a daily basis. Especially if you are following one of the low-fat eating plans described earlier, you must supplement your diet with these essential oils to help you maintain nerve health.

Minerals

"Helps build strong bodies twelve ways!" was the old slogan for Wonder Bread, the spongy white bread many of us grew up eating. The slogan referred to the twelve different vitamins and minerals that were added to enrich its nutrition-poor flour. While I certainly wouldn't encourage my patients to eat Wonder Bread, I do suggest that they supplement their diets with several minerals that are essential to bone and joint health.

Calcium, of course, is the mineral we associate most closely with our bones and teeth. But you might not know that calcium is also an important component of blood. When the blood becomes deficient in calcium (either through low consumption of calcium-rich foods or through the inability to metabolize the calcium we ingest), calcium is literally pulled out of our bones to keep the blood in balance. Loss of calcium in the bones leads to osteoporosis—weakened, brittle bones. Recent studies also seem to indicate that increased calcium intake can help prevent colon cancer as well. It's wise to take calcium in conjunction with vitamin C, which helps increase absorption. According to studies, adults need at least 1,000 mg of calcium per day (either through food sources or supplements) for optimal health.

Magnesium is often taken in conjunction with calcium as well. Essential for proper muscle function and bone growth, magnesium activates over three hundred enzymes in the body and can help protect against heart disease, stroke, and kidney stones.

Phosphorus is another important component in the makeup of our bones and teeth. We get most of our phosphorus from dietary sources such as grains.

Another mineral, *zinc,* has been shown to promote faster wound healing, boost the immune system, and maintain nervous system function. It has been used by arthritis patients to decrease joint swelling, stiffness, and other symptoms.

Other minerals needed by the body include *iron, iodine, sodium, copper, potassium,* and *selenium* (which works with vitamin E to protect the body from free-radical damage).

Many of these minerals are present in sufficient quantities in a balanced diet. However, as most of us fall far short of a balanced diet much of the time, taking a broad-range vitamin-mineral supplement is often a good idea. If you have specific health conditions that you believe might be helped by larger doses of a particular mineral, consult your health practitioner or nutritionist, who can make qualified recommendations on amounts and types of supplements to consider.

Glucosamine, Chondroitin, and Other Supplements for Healthy Joints

As we discussed in Chapter 5, each of the joints in the body (including those in the spine) is supported by a network of soft tissue—muscles, tendons, ligaments, and cartilage. As we age (or as a result of subluxation and other factors), these soft tissues sustain damage and can no longer replace themselves efficiently. When that happens, we experience pain and inflammation in the knees, hips, back, elbows, wrists, ankles, and other joints. If this wear and tear goes on long enough, the bones themselves can start to wear away, and we end up in the hospital for joint replacement surgery. Therefore, it should be clear that we want to keep the soft tissues of our joints as healthy as possible for as long as we can.

Arthritis is the catchall medical term for inflammation of the joints. It's estimated that one in seven Americans has some form of arthritis, with the incidence increasing with age. Conventional medicine has a limited number of remedies for the pain and inflammation of arthritis. While there is some emphasis on the need for regular exercise to keep joints functioning, the most common medical prescriptions for arthritis sufferers are analgesics such as acetaminophen, anti-inflammatories such as aspirin and other prescription nonsteroidal anti-inflammatories (NSAIDs), and in severe cases steroids. Unfortunately, long-term use of analgesics and NSAIDs presents significant problems, including damage to the stomach and digestive system. The only other option offered by conventional medicine is joint-replacement surgery, where the ends of the bones are replaced with plastic and metal sections designed to mimic the joint's action without pain and friction. Of course, there are significant health risks that come with any surgery, especially for older people (who are the most common patients in joint replacement). Also, these plastic and metal joints wear out over time, and a second or even third surgery may be needed if the patient lives long enough. Obviously, arthritis patients would like alternatives that don't just treat the pain and inflammation but actually heal the damage to the joints.

Chiropractic care can be of great benefit to arthritis sufferers. Chiropractic adjustments can eliminate subluxations that are associated with abnormal joint mechanics. When these subluxations are reduced, the joint can return to its normal range of motion. When nerve impulses to the joint are restored to normal, inflammation of the joint's soft tissue can be reduced or eliminated, and healing can begin. But there are also supplements that support the healing process of the soft tissue, and, specifically, the cartilage.

Chondroitin is a complex carbohydrate molecule that exists in the body's connective tissue. In cartilage, chondroitin attracts and holds fluid in the tissues. This fluid contains essential nutrients that nourish the joint's soft tissue; it also acts as a cushion, making the cartilage softer and more shock-absorbent. It is believed that chondroitin also protects the joints by strengthening cartilage's protein bonds and interacting with certain enzymes that attack connective tissue. Some very exciting evidence seems to indicate that chondroitin can actually rebuild connective tissue in some cases.

Chondroitin is often taken in conjunction with *glucosamine*. A natural sugar produced by the body, glucosamine helps produce and maintain cartilage, tendons, and ligaments. If the body doesn't produce enough glucosamine, the cartilage between the joints can dry out, crack, or wear away. Unfortunately, as we age the body produces less glucosamine. Glucosamine has been used in Europe since the 1980s to help reduce joint pain and inflammation and heal damaged joints, tendons, and ligaments. Recent studies done in Belgium attest to the efficacy of glucosamine supplements in reducing pain, allowing greater joint movement, and even decreasing damage to the joints in arthritis patients. Glucosamine is not found in food but can be produced by processing the shells of common shellfish.

Chondroitin sulfate and glucosamine sulfate (the most typical forms of these substances) are available in health food stores. Some people may experience mild digestive side effects when taking these supplements, so you may wish to take them with food. And remember, these supplements are designed not just to relieve pain but actually to rebuild cartilage, and rebuilding can take time, up to two to eight months. However, those who are committed to actually healing the body, and who want to avoid the long-term serious side effects of pain reliever and anti-inflammatory use, may wish to investigate chondroitin and glucosamine.

If you have problems with your joints, there are other nutritional supplements that can be of benefit to you—shark cartilage, MSM, and SAM-e are a few being investigated currently. However, it's always smart to consult a health care practitioner before starting any kind of supplement other than a basic multivitamin-mineral supplement. Many chiropractors have a great deal of knowledge in this area, or they will refer you to a nutritionist or naturopath.

▶ Be Practical in Choosing Your Eating Plan

For any eating plan or dietary approach to be effective, it has to be something you can follow on a regular basis with relative ease. You may do really well on a high-protein, high-fat diet, but if your spouse has a problem with it, then you may need to make some sort of accommodation. Your goal may be to eat only clean, healthy, organically grown produce, but if you're stuck on the side of the road and the only restaurant within miles is a McDonald's, you need to decide whether it's better to go hungry or to chow down on a McSalad. With eating plans or supplements—in fact, with anything concerning your health—I believe you should use common sense. Listen to the Innate Intelligence in your body. Make the healthiest choices possible, see the results, and then adjust as needed. Follow the recommendations of your health practitioners if they make sense to you, and tell them about the results you achieve.

And remember that the key to success is often to take baby steps. In nutrition, as with any other lifestyle choice, even the smallest changes—like choosing a piece of fruit instead of a candy bar for a snack, or eating fish instead of a steak, or perhaps decreasing the portion size of the steak should you choose to eat it, or eating whole-grain bread instead of white—can have a significant effect over time. Perhaps you choose to eat fish twice a week, or to take a vitamin C supplement in addition to your multivitamin. Or perhaps you decide to try a new way of eating for a week or a month in order to lose a few extra pounds. Whatever you do, just keep in mind that the goal is to allow this miracle we call the human body to function at its best by providing it with the high-quality fuel it needs.

10

Relaxation and Meditation:
Tapping a Deeper Source of Energy

There is probably no cause of suffering more prevalent in today's world than feelings of excessive stress. People from all walks of life, whether they are presidents of corporations, local police officers, or parents (and, unfortunately, their children as well), perceive their lives and our world as "stressful." Stress permeates our consciousness.

In my chiropractic practice, I see so many people laid low by the effects of stress. They walk in with lower back pain, carpal tunnel syndrome, headaches, or joint aches, or they simply feel tired all the time. "I don't know why this happened, Dr. Lenarz," they'll frequently tell me. "I didn't do anything out of the ordinary to cause this pain." After a few questions, however, I discover that they've recently lost a loved one, or they've been going through a rough patch at work or at school, or they're having problems with their spouse or children. The stress they're experiencing is having a predictable effect on the physical body. When I point this out, some patients will protest, "How can stress be causing my back to hurt?" But ongoing high levels of stress (whether physical, chemical, mental, or emotional) put the body into a habitual state of alertness that it was never designed to sustain for such long periods of time. When that happens, the body can react by creating pain or other symptoms.

Luckily, there are some simple ways to help reduce our experience of stress. Regular exercise, especially exercise such as yoga or tai chi, as described in Chapter 8, is a well-proven stress reducer. Eating a well-balanced and healthful diet, as we discussed in the last chapter, also can help you handle the everyday stresses of life. And certainly regular chiropractic care is an enormous support for the body in stressful and nonstressful situations. But one of the simplest, easiest, most available ways to reduce our experience of everyday stress is learning how to relax the mind and body through focused awareness, including meditation.

In this chapter we're going to explore how and why the body experiences stress, and, more important, how we can mitigate its negative effects. You'll also learn some simple relaxation and meditation techniques you can use anywhere, anytime, to help you handle stress and live a happier, more productive, and fulfilling life.

▶ The Biology of Stress

Not all stress is bad. In fact, stress is a vital part of our body's ability to stay alive. Much like the inherent stress designed into a structure such as a bridge to keep it standing, there are inherent physical stresses that help to keep our body erect and the walls of our blood vessels from collapsing. Even the negative experience that we call stress is actually a variation (or, more accurately, an abuse) of a lifesaving process: the fight-or-flight response. This immediate physical reaction to a perceived threat is one of the most important survival instincts we possess, and has been bred into our DNA from humankind's earliest days on the planet. But I want to explain why the fight-or-flight response can be an enemy instead of the protective instinct it was meant to be.

Suppose I'm on my evening walk and all of a sudden a large, vicious-looking dog blocks my path. The dog is growling and baring its teeth, and looks ready to leap at me in an instant. As soon as I sec the dog and perceive it as a potential threat, my body's hormone system goes into high alert. My hypothalamus, pituitary, and adrenal glands start pouring out a potent mix of steroids and neurotransmitters, including the one substance we've all learned to associate with danger: adrenaline. These chemicals produce a cascade of physical changes as I face the threat of the growling dog. My breathing becomes rapid and shallow, allowing me to take in more oxygen in case I have to flee. Blood flow increases up to 300 to 400 percent to provide my body with more energy. My digestive system shuts down almost completely (digestion is one of the most energy-consuming functions of the body, and that energy might be needed by my muscles). My immune system reacts by increasing the output of some infection- and injury-fighting cells and decreasing the output of other factors to compensate. My senses become hyperalert; my skin tingles as the blood flows to it. If I need to run, I'm ready; if the dog tries to attack me, I'm ready to fight it off. And all of this occurs within a few seconds of my seeing the dog.

This time, however, before I can run or the dog can attack, I hear a voice shouting, "Rex! Here!" The dog turns his attention away from me and bounds off across the street and into a nearby fenced yard. As soon as the threat disappears, the production of adrenaline and other hormones in my body slows. All the various systems—breathing, blood flow, digestion, and so on—that had been put on high alert start to drop back to their accustomed levels. (It takes a while for the hormones coursing through my body to dissipate.) I actually feel a sensation of relaxation when the physiological stress I was experiencing disappears. My body had done its job of protecting me by implementing the fight-or-flight response, and now it can return to its normal level of functioning.

That's the kind of stress we were designed to handle: a one-time, in-the-moment, stand-and-fight-or-run-away-from-danger response. Scientists call this *acute* stress. As a chiropractor, I frequently see people who have gone through some kind of acute stress, such as a fall or an automobile accident. Acute stress is usually followed by a short period of recovery time when the body regains its equilibrium. However, the kind of stress most people complain of isn't the acute variety; rather, it's ongoing or *chronic* stress. Chronic stress occurs when we are subjected to consistent stressful situations that cause the arousal of the fight-or-flight response. Hormones flow through the body, causing all the physiological changes described earlier; however, because the stress either does not go away or isn't extreme enough to cause us actually to have to run or fight, we never get to relax. The urge to fight or flee is suppressed, but the hormones keep flowing anyway. Our bodies have little or no time to recuperate, and we end up in a constant state of low-level adrenal arousal. Eventually, the adrenals and other hormone-producing glands become exhausted, and we experience fatigue, illness, and a general sense of malaise.

But adrenal exhaustion affects a lot more than just the glands. All the body systems most directly affected by adrenal overload— the heart, digestion, and nerves—are also in chronic states of either over- or underutilization. Over time, this can result in small to significant damage to these systems, and all sorts of health problems can arise as a result. For example:

- Many of the physiological effects of stress put huge demands on the heart and cardiovascular system; therefore, stress is a major trigger for angina (heart pain). Chronic stress can contribute to heart rhythm abnormalities and raise the likelihood of heart attacks. It can also be a factor in the possibility of stroke.

- While fight-or-flight stress increases immune system activity in the short term, *chronic* stress wears down and eventually suppresses the body's natural immune function, creating a greater risk of infection and/or illness.

- Because stress hormones literally stop the body's digestive processes from proceeding normally, it's no surprise that flare-ups in peptic ulcers and inflammatory bowel disease are common by-products of chronic stress.

- Chronic stress is associated with the development of insulin resistance, which is a primary factor in the development of adult-onset diabetes.

- Stress can produce increased pain in people with arthritis and other joint problems, including carpal tunnel syndrome.

- Back pain is one of the more common complaints tied to stress.

- Headaches, especially tension-type headaches, are clearly linked to stressful events. In this case, stress is translated by the body into muscle and blood vessel contractions, thus producing the headache. Some research shows that stress can be a contributing factor in migraines as well.

- Stress can cause sleep disturbances and sexual dysfunction.

- Stress can have a significant effect on concentration, memory, and learning.

- Stress exacerbates many allergic reactions, especially skin conditions like hives, psoriasis, acne, rosacea, and eczema.

- Stress leads to self-medication through drugs, alcohol, tobacco, abnormal eating habits, television, and so on.

- Stress can affect appetite. Some people may stop eating, or overindulge in specific kinds of foods. Salt, sugar, or fat cravings are common responses to chronic stress. (What we call "comfort foods"—mashed potatoes, soups, breads, carbohydrates, desserts, and so on—satisfy stress cravings; they are relatively easy to digest and produce a feeling of fullness in the stomach.)

- Severe stress is commonly associated with onset of depression or anxiety.

- Stress can have a direct and powerful effect on subluxations. Although most subluxations initially come from trauma, stress is a major player in keeping them in existence. Remember, a subluxation is not just a misalignment of a bone but also an inflammation of the surrounding soft tissue, which includes muscles, cartilage, joints, and tendons. When a patient is under chronic stress, the hormones and neurotransmitters that are being overproduced can continue the cycle of inflammation even if the subluxation has been reduced by an adjustment. Conversely, when someone eliminates chronic stress, the healing process that is initiated when the subluxation is adjusted can take its natural course; inflammation disappears, and the soft tissues can start to return to normal.

Stress not only can make people sick, but also can be a major contributing factor in death. Several years ago, a psychiatrist at the University of Rochester investigated 160 cases of sudden death that had no specific physical cause or explanation. Of those deaths, 58 percent occurred when the deceased was bereaved, in mourning, or had experienced some other serious loss. Thirty-five percent occurred in those who were experiencing some kind of threat. Only 6 percent of the sudden deaths occurred during what the psychiatrist termed a "time of pleasure." And of course, it's also well documented that more heart attacks occur on Monday morning than at any other time of the week—right when most people are returning to work! Excessive stress can damage our health as well as our mental and emotional well-being. We need to learn how to decrease our stress if possible, and develop a wide range of strategies to manage stress no matter what its origin.

▶ Physical, Mental, and Emotional Stress

Our bodies *need* stress—not just to get us out of danger, but also to be healthy. Physical stress is what causes our bones to strengthen and our muscles to grow. Whenever you move, you are putting stress on certain parts of your body. When you exercise, you are definitely placing greater stress on different bones and muscle groups. Fighting against physical stress—indeed, fighting against the effects of gravity—produces increased health. So a certain amount of stress is one of the conditions of life.

This physiological necessity has proved a huge problem for astronauts who spend long periods of time in space. When they are in space, they work and live in conditions of low or no gravity. There is nothing for the muscles to work against; little or no physical effort has to be expended for even the most arduous physical tasks. As a result, muscles start to shrink and bones begin to thin. In a matter of weeks the body begins to deteriorate, simply because there *is* no physical stress. The same process occurs if you break a leg or an arm, or have to stay in bed for a prolonged period of time. Your muscles shrink, and you become physically weaker.

Children are under biological stress constantly—it's called growing. Puberty is nothing but a series of hormonal, physical, and biological stresses. A woman goes through biological stress as part of her monthly hormonal cycle, let alone the stresses of pregnancy, birth, and menopause. Every time you get sick with anything—from a cold to the worst of infection—you are experiencing biological stress.

Luckily, the body is designed to handle most physical and biological stress quickly, easily, and efficiently. But as almost everyone knows from personal experience, what most of us call stress has very little to do with physical or biological events and a lot more to do with our minds and emotions. Mental and emotional factors create more chronic stress than physical ones ever do. How many people do I see in my office who have suffered some physical trauma, such as an auto accident, but whose suffering is mainly caused by the emotional fallout from the accident!

Pain from *acute* stress can create the mental and emotional problems that then produce the condition of *chronic* stress. For example, I recently encountered a former patient of mine who was in a car accident about a year ago. He had had some back problems before, but the accident caused him ongoing pain that hadn't been resolved. He also hadn't kept up with his chiropractic care, so now he's in pain every day. Unfortunately, he has to work, although time off would help him heal. He needs to earn money for his family, but because of his discomfort he can't do his job the way he'd like to. As a result, his boss doesn't give him the responsibility he used to have. My former patient is stressed by the pain and by the possibility of losing his job and the financial difficulties that would present.

He's also experiencing mental and emotional stress in his relationships. Especially with back pain, since there is no visible indication of your internal experience, people don't think of you as disabled or stressed (unless they've experienced chronic pain themselves at some point). Often others can't understand why you're so "cranky" or "difficult," even though you think you're doing your best to cope with a body that seems to have turned against you. Pain creates tensions in relationships, in job situations, as well as the basic physical stress of dealing with pain, and the mental and emotional stress makes the physical stress much, much worse.

Study after study has shown that many neuromuscular conditions are caused or exacerbated by mental and emotional stress. TMJ, or temporomandibular joint pain, is one such condition; the joint between the jawbone and the skull hurts, often because of unconscious clenching or grinding of the teeth. Typically back, neck, and other musculoskeletal problems may originate in some kind of physical stress, such as an accident, fall, or abnormal motion over time, but mental and emotional stress will cause the conditions to flare up or worsen. I see patients all the time who do well under chiropractic care but have some permanent tissue damage surrounding a particular vertebra or joint. The damage rarely bothers them—they can participate in sports and do heavy yard work—but if they get into an argument with their spouse, out the back goes. Some researchers theorize that stress has a greater impact on those areas or systems where someone already has an inherent weakness of some kind. If, for example, you are prone to a sensitive stomach, that's the first place your body will react when it's under stress. If you have bad knees, or were in an accident as a child and hurt your back, whenever things get overly stressful your knees or back will "go out." And usually the stress that produces these effects is mental and emotional rather than physical.

With most mental and emotional stress, the *circumstances* causing the stress are less important than our *perception* of those circumstances. I have patients who sleep until ten every morning, work part-time, and are totally stressed out. I have other patients who work twelve-hour days and take care of a family to boot, and they are happy as can be. Their stress levels are very low simply because they perceive and respond to their conditions in a very different way. *Stress is not something that happens to us; it is the way we respond to what is happening around us.*

This is not to say that we're to blame for our stress. Sometimes stress is a very appropriate and natural response to our circumstances. Losing a job is often stressful. Grief over the death of a loved one is very stressful. Divorce or breaking up a relationship is usually stressful. Caring for a new baby is extremely stressful physically for the parents. But we should still accept that our stress is produced by our response to the situation, not the situation itself. And if we get appropriate support for ourselves physically, mentally, and emotionally, we can change our response and decrease or eliminate the toxic impact of stress.

Like all healing, dealing with stress is part of a cycle. We experience an event—whether it is a physical or emotional trauma or just an ongoing challenge to our well-being—and we create physical, mental, and emotional responses to it. Those responses can be short-lived, that is, acute stress followed by a quick recovery of our equilibrium, or long-lasting, as the body spirals downward in a cycle of chronic physical stress exacerbated by our negative emotional and mental patterns.

But the good news is that we can intervene at any point in that cycle and cause the body to spiral upward to health instead of downward to disease. The intervention can be physical (such as chiropractic care, massage, rest, exercise, and so on), mental (applying any of the focusing and relaxing techniques you'll find in this chapter), or emotional (talking things out with friends, or perhaps seeking professional counseling). Any positive intervention can affect your stress levels dramatically, allowing your body's natural processes to complete the needed healing. When that happens, your health can be regained and maintained even if the circumstances that caused your stress haven't changed. Consider the difference between a stressed mother and a relaxed one when faced with a whining child. The stressed mom is far more likely to snap at her child; however, while the relaxed mom may still be annoyed by the behavior, she's probably going to be able to hold her temper and deal with the child in a more resourceful fashion.

No one can be relaxed all the time. Just as stress is a part of life, processing stress is one of the most important parts of health. The best thing that we can do to stay healthy is to develop an array of techniques, tools, and strategies for dealing with stress *before* it hits us between the eyes and saps our vitality and energy. If we can learn to recognize the causes of our stress—whether we face a physical challenge like pain, or if most of our problem is due to mental or emotional challenges—we can choose very specific remedies to interrupt the cycle and put us back on the road to health.

▶ Relaxation and Stress Reduction: Physical Support

Many of us handle stress by engaging in activities that are harmful. We may go straight for sugary, fat-laden comfort foods that turn us into couch potatoes, distracted for hours with TV; we may take a little too much alcohol to take the edge off, or use (and perhaps overuse) both legal and illegal drugs. But all of these strategies for getting out of stress don't work in the long term because they are detrimental to our health, lowering our stamina and decreasing our ability to deal with stress in the long term. However, there are also many simple, constructive ways you can lower your physical stress by supporting your body rather than abusing it. Here are just a few.

Diet—Eating for Health *and* Comfort

When the body is under stress, the physical demands placed upon every system are enormous, and therefore the need for high-quality nutrition is even greater. Unfortunately, stress can also cause the digestive system to slow down or stop working altogether—quite a dilemma. You can assist your body to receive optimal levels of nutrition by doing three things. First, make your mealtimes as calm and supportive as possible. Don't eat at your desk at work, or while you're feeding your children. Take time to sit down and eat slowly and calmly. I find taking a few deep breaths before I start to eat helps me to leave the rest of my day behind and focus on my meal. If eating with friends is a pleasurable experience for you, then do so; if eating alone is better for you, dine by yourself. And although I may risk sounding like your mother, concentrate on chewing your food thoroughly. A great deal of digestion begins in the mouth, when the chemicals in saliva combine with the physical breaking up of food by chewing.

Second, choose foods that support you nutritionally and won't upset your digestion. This may mean avoiding many of the foods you are craving— high-sugar, high-salt, high-fat, low-nutrition processed snacks. Of course, you can eat sugar, salt, and fats in moderation, but remember that the goal of food is to support the body first and the emotions second. Continue to drink plenty of water and to eat healthfully, choosing from a range of fruits, vegetables, grains, proteins, healthy fats, and so on. If you feel a need for comfort food, try things like oatmeal with a little brown sugar, popcorn (the real stuff, not the oversalted kind in the microwavable bags), cooked fruits, and so on. Many of us have foods that our mothers gave us when we were sick as kids. Usually those foods were moderately healthy, and we associated them with a feeling of being taken care of, so you might want to take care of yourself by eating them again.

Third, look at the vitamins and nutritional supplements you are currently taking. You may want to adjust the amounts to give yourself some additional support. For example, because stress can lower resistance to infection, you might want to increase your vitamin C. I do recommend, however, that you consult a nutritionist or health care professional before you take large doses of any supplement.

Fourth, don't increase your consumption of alcohol and caffeine. Many of us think that the coffee and drinks we consume will help us unwind, but in truth these substances put even greater stress on the body. Moderation is the key. A cup of coffee or a glass of wine probably won't cause a problem; drinking coffee all night or downing the entire bottle of wine most definitely will.

Rest—Let Your Body Recover

Most of us have been kept awake at various times by pain, worry, or upset, so we know that stress can interfere with the body's natural sleep patterns. And since we tend to be inadequately rested anyway (over 40 percent of adults in the United States report they are so sleepy at times that it interferes with their daily activities), stress just exacerbates what is already a problem.

Getting enough restful, deep sleep is an important way to support yourself in times of stress. Make sure you allow enough time to get the sleep you need. While most adults require around eight hours of sleep a night, some people need more to feel adequately rested. And because stress depletes so many of our biological systems, we may need even more rest than usual to allow our bodies to recuperate. The key is to get rest*ful* rather than rest*less* sleep. Avoid caffeine or other stimulants for at least six hours before bedtime. Don't exercise late in the day, as this can cause wakefulness. (However, including exercise as part of your daily regimen promotes more restful sleep. Try exercising early in the morning, or during your lunch hour.) Finish your last meal of the day before 8 P.M. to give your digestive system adequate rest, too. Create a sleep environment that's quiet, dark, and slightly cool.

If you are having temporary difficulties falling asleep, try some natural remedies. A warm bath, hot milk, even some gentle massage can help you glide into the restful state that leads to sleep. You can also try some natural supplements: melatonin (the hormone that triggers sleepiness), valerian, and chamomile tea have all been proven to aid sleep. You can also try some relaxation exercises (see Chapter 8) to help you release any physical tension before you go to bed. I also have a friend who recommends leaving all your worries and tensions outside of the bedroom before bedtime. He makes a ritual of stopping at the bedroom door and mentally piling all his worries beside the door frame. "I know they'll be there when I get up," he says. "But this way I don't have to take them to bed with me."

Exercise—the Body's Natural Tranquilizer

As we discussed in Chapter 8, exercise provides a cornucopia of benefits for our physical, mental, and emotional well-being. By definition, exercise places demands (stress) on the body, strengthening the muscles, bones, and cardiovascular system. People who exercise regularly experience far fewer of the physical effects of stress, simply because their bodies are stronger, in better shape, and more able to cope with a higher level of demand.

But there are other stress-reduction benefits to regular exercise. For most people, exercise can be a welcome break from stressful situations. It can distract us by causing us to focus on physical activity rather than our troubles. Those who exercise regularly often feel more in control of their lives (or at least, of this one area). And strenuous exercise can produce the same kind of relaxation response that people experience after acute stress subsides.

If you already have a regular exercise program, now is the time to keep to it faithfully. Continue to go to the gym, head out for a walk, go for a swim, or take an aerobics or yoga class. If you have started doing the yoga or tai chi exercises described in Chapter 8, continue with them. If you feel up to it, you can increase the intensity and/or frequency of your workouts. But remember, exercise should decrease rather than increase your stress level. Someone who has been going to one aerobics class a week and starts going four times a week when under stress may become physically exhausted—and therefore less able to handle mental and emotional stress. Use your exercise as a means of getting away from it all rather than as another way to burn out.

If you are not exercising regularly, you can certainly begin a regular exercise program even when you're experiencing stress. You'll gain all of the benefits listed above—as long as you don't overdo it. Start small; try ten minutes of exercise three times a week, and gradually build up to thirty minutes or more every other day. And be sure to check with your health care professional before you begin any kind of exercise.

In times of stress, I highly recommend the yoga exercises described in Chapter 8. Not only will they help support you physically, but yoga also is proven to decrease anxiety, lower high blood pressure, help with asthma, and decrease the severity of tension-related problems such as headache or backache. It also elevates mood and improves concentration and ability to focus.

For quick tension release anytime, anywhere, try the following: Stand with your feet together and your hands by your sides. Imagine a string coming up through your body, stretching from your heels to your back and then out of the top of your head. Then imagine there is someone pulling gently on the string, causing your entire body to stretch gently upward. Feel your spine and neck gently elongating upward while you keep your feet planted on the ground. Now, imagine that the string goes slack, causing your head and upper body to come forward. Allow yourself to bend at the waist, your head hanging loosely, your hands and arms flopping down toward the floor. Feel all the tension draining from your fingertips. Then allow yourself to come up slowly, stacking one vertebra on top of the other. Your head is the last thing to come up, and it rests comfortably on top of the neck.

Massage

Massage is one of the most effective—and often overlooked—tools for reducing tension and allowing the body to release stress. If you've ever had a sore muscle and rubbed it, or had a friend give you a neck, shoulder, or back rub when you're experiencing discomfort in those areas, you know the benefits of massage. Massage not only eases soreness and eliminates tension, but it also has been shown to slow the heart rate while producing a state of increased yet relaxed alertness.

Massage helps us release tension in three ways. First, rubbing a sore muscle increases circulation and lymph flow to that particular area of the body. This promotes healing by carrying away from the area the biochemical residue of the microscopic damage that caused the soreness in the first place, and replacing it with healing chemicals. Second, the heat generated by massage helps the muscle fibers and connective tissue to stretch and loosen, allowing them to return to their normal degree of extension. Third (and this is a trait that massage and chiropractic share), human touch has been proven to have healing properties not strictly accounted for by biology. The tactile sense that someone is caring for our physical well-being is a powerful component in the healing process, and massage taps into this sense.

There are many types of massage to choose from: Swedish (which is the kind most of us are familiar with, where the muscles are rubbed and manipulated), shiatsu (which works with the meridians in the body to release blocked energy and restore normal flow and function), acupressure, Rolfing, reflexology (which works primarily with acupuncture points in the hands and feet), and so on. If you are interested in massage, your chiropractor or other alternative health care provider may be able to recommend a good massage therapist. Many health clubs and spas have massage therapists on staff. In many states, massage therapists must receive a certain amount of training and be licensed to work on patients, so it's perfectly acceptable to ask massage therapists about the kind of training they received and what kind of license they have.

When you get a massage, make sure you are comfortable with both the therapist and the type of massage you are getting. Remember, the goal of massage is the release of tension and reduction of stress, so it's important for you to trust your therapist enough to relax and put yourself into his or her hands.

Chiropractic Care

Reducing or eliminating the effects of any kind of stress is one of the great benefits of regular chiropractic care. Various studies have documented that immediately after an adjustment, many people experience a relaxation response. It's as if the body has been holding on to tension in preparation for fight or flight, and the adjustment breaks that physical lock, allowing the body to relax back to its normal, natural, healthful state.

Chiropractic can help ease the effects of both acute and chronic stress. If someone has been in an accident, for instance, a series of adjustments can help put the body back to rights, reducing and eventually eliminating the causes of pain, and therefore one of the major causes of stress. But chiropractic can also help ease the mental and emotional reactions to acute trauma. Chronic pain itself creates a fight-or-flight response, accompanied by anxiety and aggressiveness. If people are in pain, it's also difficult for them to relax. It's as if the body ties itself into knots in the act of coping with chronic pain. Luckily, regular chiropractic care can help ease this chronic pain, by returning the body to its normal range of motion and triggering the relaxation response on a regular basis. But more than that, chiropractic care is founded on the principle of mind, body, and emotions being part of the same organism. If you reduce the level of physical stress—through elimination of pain and triggering of the relaxation response—then mental and emotional stress will be reduced as well.

For instance, say you have been in an automobile accident. You experienced some physical trauma to your neck (whiplash) and you're in pain. Because the accident kept you away from work for a week, you're worried about your job. You're also concerned because your spouse was in the car and he or she isn't feeling too well, either. You're trying to support your spouse emotionally while handling your own pain, as well as all the details of dealing with insurance companies, police reports, checking in with your boss while you're away from the office, and so on. You're feeling stress physically, mentally, and emotionally. You decide you need some stress relief, so you do some of the things listed in this chapter—you get more rest, you support yourself nutritionally, you do a few of the relaxation and focus exercises we'll talk about later. But without chiropractic care, you're fighting an uphill battle. The physical stress caused by the accident and the subsequent mental and emotional stress are locked into your body; chiropractic care can help you break that lock.

Say you finally decide to go to a chiropractor. With a few adjustments, the pain in your neck and back is reduced or eliminated as the spine is allowed to return to normal functioning. The stress you were experiencing from dealing with chronic pain decreases—benefit number one. That has an impact on your mental and emotional state—benefit number two. You find yourself able to rest better; you can exercise again without discomfort; you may even find your digestion improves—more benefits. As you continue to use some of the relaxation techniques in this chapter, you discover their effects are increased simply because your brain and your body are "talking" to one another again—more benefits. Simply put, chiropractic care not only can help decrease stress, but also can increase the effectiveness of other stress-reducing strategies you may choose to employ.

I have listed chiropractic care under the category of physical support for stress reduction and relaxation, but as I hope you see, it really serves as the bridge between physical and mental and emotional support. Regular visits to your chiropractor can be of enormous help in dealing with acute or chronic stress and restoring yourself to radiant health and vitality.

▶ Mental and Emotional Relaxation

Mental and emotional stress are based on our perception of events rather than on the events themselves. We see this happen all the time: The project at work that you regard as an opportunity is for your colleague a test that she's afraid she'll fail. The annual piano recital is a trauma for your son but a snap for your daughter. The stress we experience is either mitigated or exacerbated by our perceptions, and if we change our perceptions, the stress we are experiencing will change as well.

So the first step in reducing stress is to ask yourself "Why am I stressed?" Is there another way you can view this situation that will put it in a more positive, healthful light? Other questions to ask: "What's a different way of looking at this?" "How is this an opportunity?" "What can I learn from this that will help me in the future?" "What's funny about this?" (Humor is a great way of diffusing or eliminating stress.) "Will this even matter ten years from now?"

Another great way to reduce mental and emotional stress is to talk about the situation with a friend, preferably one who can provide a different perspective. Don't seek out someone who's just going to reinforce your own bad feelings. We all know well-meaning people who are great at commiserating with us and make us feel better simply because they're willing to listen. But sometimes we need more than commiseration. Seek out the folks who not only will listen to you, but also will provide an alternative view of your problems and ideas for solutions. That's the value of most professional counselors. They're not there to agree about how you were wronged but to apply their expertise to help you resolve problems and create changes that will support you in living a healthier, happier life. I believe it's important to seek the help and counsel of professional therapists if you believe it will be of assistance in your particular circumstances.

Sometimes the best thing you can do to lower your stress is to take a mental and emotional break from your circumstances. New parents know the value of this; for a new mom, the opportunity to take a shower or bath while someone else watches the baby can feel like a week in the Caribbean! Make time for yourself when you're stressed. Keep your commitment to regular exercise. Go out for lunch instead of eating at your desk. Listen to a great piece of music. I knew a woman who worked at a very stressful job as a customer service associate. She was on the phone eight hours a day handling people's complaints, but every hour on the hour she would get up from her desk, put on her Walkman earphones, and dance around her cubicle to her favorite Michael Jackson music. Whatever you choose to do, make sure your activity is something you enjoy that takes your mind off whatever is stressing you out.

While breaks can help you reduce physical, mental, and emotional stress, the key to relaxing the mind is often as simple as changing what you're focusing on. Relaxation and meditation are simply a matter of focused awareness: focusing on something that produces feelings of calm, peace, and tranquility rather than worry. Have you ever been worried about something, or in pain, and all of a sudden you see a beautiful sunset, or someone you love but haven't seen in a long time walks into the room? For a moment your worries or pains are gone. You're concentrating on the beauty of nature or on your unexpected visitor. Simply by changing what you focus on, your stress has disappeared in an instant.

The key with these relaxation techniques is to bypass the mind's tendency to keep itself busy with thought. For most of us, the mind is like an untrained puppy, running from one thing to another, peeing in the corners or chewing up the furniture, creating chaos because it has no direction. Most of the time we let our minds run amok.

In the pages that follow, I'm going to give examples of how to focus your attention consciously, to eliminate stress and encourage relaxation. There are dozens of ways to do this, and below I've described some of my personal favorites. All of them are very easy and pleasurable; you just have to set aside a few moments to do them. But remember, the key to success in changing your life is to take baby steps, and acknowledge your successes along the way. In my practice I've noticed that some very stressed people seem to think that learning to relax is more stressful than continuing to be stressed! These techniques are very simple, but they can take you from chronic stress to regular relaxation.

Technique #1: Practice the Yoga Breath

Remember the yoga breath in Chapter 8? There you were focusing on allowing the breath to arise from your abdomen, then your chest, and finally your shoulders. In order to breathe that way, however, you had to pay attention to your breath. You can use the same attention to the breath to relax yourself. Just close your eyes and turn your attention to the place your breath is arising from. Take a slow, deep breath in, and then breathe out, focusing on how the breath leaves the body naturally. Within a very few breaths, you'll find yourself relaxing. Several full yoga breaths for fifteen minutes in a seated position is one of the easiest ways to focus the mind while letting the body take a "breather"—literally.

Technique #2: Focus on Your Body

If you've ever been through Lamaze childbirth training or you've seen it depicted in movies or on TV, you might remember how women are taught to breathe in different patterns during different parts of labor. This not only helps their bodies by providing extra oxygen, but, more important, it allows them to focus on something other than the pain. Putting your focus on tensing and relaxing the body sequentially can help both your muscles and your mind to let go.

Try this exercise. Lie down on the floor, preferably on a carpeted surface or on a mat of some kind. Your legs and arms should not be crossed. Begin by tensing the muscles in your toes and feet as much as possible. Hold the tension for a count of five, until you can feel the muscles tensing completely, then immediately let them relax utterly. Your muscles should feel heavy and totally relaxed. Do the same thing with the ankles, calf muscles, knees, thigh muscles, buttock muscles, pelvis, and chest, tensing each set of muscles completely and then letting them go. Then, starting with your fingers, tense the fingers, hands, arms, shoulders, and neck in sequence, tensing each set of muscles and then letting them go. When you get to your head, tense the jaw muscles, the eyes, the forehead, and the scalp in order, letting each group of muscles go in turn. Keep breathing deeply throughout the entire exercise.

After you've reached the top of your head, breathe gently for a few minutes. Check to see if there is any tension remaining in any part of your body. If so, tense that part of the body to its utmost and then let it go. You should feel like a rag doll someone has thrown on the floor. Relax in this position for at least ten minutes.

Technique #3: Focus on Nature

Another friend of mine worked in a very hectic office on the top floor of a ten-story office building in San Diego, California. The office had wall-to-wall glass windows facing west, and especially during the winter, the sunsets were gorgeous. Every day she would check to see what time sunset would happen, and at that time she'd walk around announcing, "Sunset break!" to her co-workers. Everyone would stop and gather by the windows, watching the reds, oranges, golds, and purples fill the sky as the sun sank into the Pacific Ocean.

Nature is one of the most healing and relaxing forces available to us. Yet with the busyness of today's world, we often fail to notice its miracles. Relax your mind and feed your thirst for beauty by spending a few moments in nature, appreciating its wonder. Sit by a body of water. Stroll through a park or a garden. Mow your lawn or work in the yard (but only if you enjoy doing so). Listen to the sounds of the birds in the trees. Even in the most concrete-filled cities, there is something you can appreciate—a blue sky or the clouds racing past, the feel of rain or the sound of a water fountain. Even a tree or a plant can help you connect to the nurturing force of nature's beauty.

Technique #4: Focus on the Present Moment

Someone once said that stress often arises when we're thinking about either the past or the future, but rarely when we're focusing on the present. We're stressed because of an action we've taken in the past, or past problems in a relationship, or an old injury or accident. Even more likely, we're worrying about something that hasn't happened yet and may never occur! (By definition, worry is about something in the future.) On the other hand, almost anytime we're fully in the present moment, focused only on what we're doing or feeling, we are a lot less likely to be stressed.

Look at very young children—they live almost completely in the present moment. By putting your focus exclusively on the present moment, on whatever task, person, communication, or sensory object that is before you, you'll find that it's a lot more difficult to experience worry or regret.

There is an easy exercise called "simple seeing" based on this practice of experiencing the present moment. Choose an object, preferably one of some kind of beauty—a lit candle, a flower or a plant, a favorite item on your desk that has some pleasurable meaning for you are examples. Now, focus your attention on the object. Your effort should be simply to observe the object. Don't name it, don't think about it, don't catalogue its characteristics, don't try to create a meaning or make up a story about it; simply look at the object, observing it as it is. Allow your mind to focus only on the object for five minutes. At the end of that time, notice your mental and emotional state. Most people find this an excellent technique for focusing the mind and calming the emotions.

Focusing on the present moment is valuable in relationships, too. Far too often we create conversations in our heads instead of being present with the person we're with. Practice focusing all your attention and awareness on the other person. Really hear what he or she has to say. Watch the body language, listen to the tone of voice, let them finish a thought before you come up with a response. You'll be amazed how much deeper your conversations will feel, and how happy people are when they feel they are truly being heard. Being in the present moment and truly giving your attention to someone else is the best gift you will ever bestow on the people you love.

Technique #5: Focus on Someone or Something You Love

Have you ever been happily in love? What's it like to focus your mind and emotions on the person you care for? What's your stress level? If the love is reciprocated, most of the time thinking about the beloved makes us feel wonderful. In a similar way, if you have something you absolutely love to do, simply thinking about that pastime is almost like taking a mini-vacation in the middle of your daily activities.

If you're experiencing stress at work, put pictures of your loved ones on your desk. It's even better if the pictures are of a happy time you spent together—a vacation, a school recital, a honeymoon, and so on. When those moments of stress occur, look at your pictures and remember that time. Ask yourself questions like "How'd I get so lucky to have such a great wife/husband/boyfriend/ girlfriend/kids/parents/friends?" Or put reminders of your favorite pastime in your office. Put your softball glove in the corner, hang up a poster from the community-theater play you acted in, or post a great photo of skiing or snowboarding or surfing or golfing or whatever your favorite sport is. Take a few moments out of your day to imagine yourself doing your favorite activity. And allow yourself a smile while you do it!

Technique #6: Focus on a Word, Phrase, or Prayer

While this technique overlaps with meditation (which we'll discuss next), it can also be a very simple and effective means for concentrating the mind. You choose a word, phrase, or even a prayer and repeat it over and over again, either silently or out loud.

Almost every religious tradition uses this technique to help quiet the mind and focus it on something higher. Catholics pray the rosary, repeating a sequence of prayers a certain number of times. Jews have prayers in Hebrew that are repeated for different occasions. Muslims pray five times a day, repeating specific prayers each time. Many Hindus use the syllable *om*, which they regard as the sound from which the universe was born. Other traditions have specific phrases or prayers that are said over and over again.

In 1968, Dr. Herbert Benson of Harvard University was asked to study the effects of Transcendental Meditation on longtime meditators. He documented the relaxation response that was produced in these meditators as a result of their practice. He also discovered that the word or syllable chosen as a focus didn't matter; the same relaxation response could be produced if a subject repeated the word *one* over and over again. Nowadays many doctors prescribe this mental relaxation technique for patients with high blood pressure or other stress-related illnesses.

To use this technique yourself, choose a word or phrase that has meaning for you. (In truth, you can use any word, but many people find it easier and more pleasant to focus on something they like.) Sit comfortably, close your eyes, and repeat the word or phrase to yourself silently. It's helpful if you repeat it in time with your breath: Breathe in and say the word or phrase, breathe out and say it. Do this for a period of five minutes at first, and then increase the time gradually until you reach fifteen to twenty minutes.

▶ Meditation: A Proven Means of Stress Reduction

If you want to take your relaxation further, I strongly recommend creating a regular time for meditation in your day. As I said earlier, meditation is simply focusing the mind on one word, thought, breath, object, and so on, and letting all other distractions disappear. While earlier generations regarded meditation as something practiced only by Eastern mystics, nowadays it is almost part of the mainstream.

Medical studies over the past thirty years have documented many different health benefits to regular meditation.

- Meditators live longer and report they experience a better quality of life than other people.

- Meditators generally make less use of the health care system, simply because they are healthier.

- When practiced regularly, meditation seems to reduce chronic pain in many patients.

- Meditators report less anxiety. Long-term meditators tend to have stronger psychological coping mechanisms than average.

- Meditation can produce a reduction of high blood pressure and in serum cholesterol levels.

- Substance abusers are helped by regular meditation. Meditation has also been proven helpful in the treatment of post-traumatic stress syndrome in Vietnam veterans.

- Meditation seems to help lower blood cortisol and adrenaline levels brought on by stress. The practiced meditator can achieve a reduction in heart rate, blood pressure, adrenaline levels, and skin temperature while meditating.

- Meditation even seems to increase scores on some intelligence-related measuring systems.

Meditation fits very nicely within the philosophical basis of chiropractic. B. J. Palmer often referred to the value of "getting in touch with our Innate," the Innate Intelligence that makes our bodies work and allows us to move, think, and feel. If there is indeed a vast wisdom that lies within us, something infinite, what value could that have in our lives? And how can we get in touch with it? One of the simplest ways is through meditation.

How do you meditate? There are many ways to do so; several of them you already learned in the relaxation techniques we discussed above. There are three simple keys to basic meditation.

1. Make sure your body is relaxed. Sit in a comfortable position, with your back straight. You should be able to sit comfortably in this position for at least fifteen minutes. Prop yourself up with pillows if you need to do so to be comfortable. If you choose, you can lie down, but meditating is

different from sleeping. Don't make yourself so comfortable that you're going to drop off.

2. Choose something you will focus on during your meditation. You can focus on your breath; you can focus on your body; you can focus on a word, a prayer, a phrase; you can focus on an object such as a lit candle. The idea is to point the mind toward one thing. You can close your eyes or keep them open, as long as the mind continues to remain on your chosen focus: object/word/breath, etc.

3. Especially when you first start meditating, it's natural for thoughts and distractions to arise. Don't worry about it; simply notice them without emotion, and bring your attention back to the focus of your meditation. If it helps, think of your thoughts as clouds passing through the sky, and focus on the blue sky that is always there.

The key to experiencing the greatest benefits of meditation seems to be practicing it regularly. You can start with as little as five minutes and increase your time until you reach fifteen to twenty minutes a session. Many practiced meditators recommend meditating for twenty minutes both first thing in the morning and again in the early evening. But whatever you choose to do, try to meditate every day. You'll discover the cumulative stress reduction benefits are well worth the investment of your time.

There are actually a number of different meditation techniques you can use to expand your experience of meditation. Walking meditation, where you repeat a word or phrase rhythmically as you walk, can increase the relaxation benefits you experience from this form of exercise. Meditation is often featured as a component of various yoga schools; again, linking the focus of the mind to the discipline of the body makes each more powerful. If you are interested in exploring meditation further, there are a number of places where you can learn different meditation techniques. Transcendental Meditation is one of the most popular forms, and you can find TM teachers in many cities and towns throughout the United

States. Yoga instructors often teach meditation as part of their discipline; if you have a yoga teacher, check with him or her. You can also find alternative health care practitioners who can teach you the basics of meditation.

Remember, the goal with any kind of relaxation is to let go, not to do it perfectly. I see far too many Type-A personalities come into my office and ask me, "Dr. Lenarz, I started meditating and such-and-such happened. Am I doing this right?" Relaxation and meditation aren't about "doing it right"; they're about allowing the mind, body, and emotions to return to their normal, healthy, relaxed state. If you're worried about being perfect, then all you're doing is stressing about relaxing, and that's pretty counterproductive. So forget about the results. Just pick something that's simple and that you will enjoy. You can choose something physical, such as chiropractic care or massage; you can take an emotional break from whatever's causing you stress by talking to a friend; or you can relax your mind through any of the focusing and meditation techniques listed here.

Since stress is caused by physical, mental, and emotional factors, you can decrease it by using physical, mental, or emotional solutions. Stress relief in any area will affect the other two in a positive way. Indeed, there have been studies indicating that a combination of stress relief techniques produces the greatest effect. In one such study of children and adolescents with depression and adjustment disorders, combining yoga, massage, and the muscle relaxation/focus technique I described earlier reduced both feelings of anxiety and levels of stress hormones.

One final point: You don't have to wait until you are experiencing high levels of stress to use the techniques in this chapter. Learning to focus the mind, to take care of your physical body, and to get the emotional support you need before things get really tough are all critical coping skills that will help you live a healthier, relaxed, more vibrant life. So kill the monster while it's little, as a friend of mine says. Take care of your stress before it's severe enough to cause you physical, mental, or emotional pain. You'll make your life happier, and probably live longer as a result.

11

Enjoying Good Health:
The Process of a Lifetime

Somewhere around the sixteenth or seventeenth century, scientists started describing the human body as a machine. Muscles were likened to pulleys, bones to the timbers that held up a building, the heart to a pump, the lungs to a pair of bellows, the stomach to a furnace. This mind-set has affected the perception of the body in Western society to this very day. It underlies the unstated but immensely powerful belief that the human body can be repaired in the same way you would fix a machine. Once you've figured out what's wrong with a machine, it's usually a pretty simple task to repair it. Pull out a component that's not working and replace it with one that does, and bingo! The machine runs perfectly. Lubricate the moving parts, or fix a cog that's out of alignment, and everything goes back to the way it was when the machine first started operating. Sometimes all you have to do is hit the reset button and the machine will return to its original operating instructions, eliminating any glitches that might have occurred since then.

In some ways, it would be great if the human body were like a machine—but it most definitely is *not*. The human body is a conglomeration of intricate, interconnected biological processes; it resembles a plant or a tree more than it does a machine. As we've seen with organ transplants, we can't just pull a component out of a human body and replace it; when we try to do so, we have to take hundreds of different biological and chemical consequences into account. And while you can "lubricate the joints" of the body with good nutrition, supplements, and even drugs, there may be many complicated unintended consequences with every intervention you make.

When it comes to chiropractic care, even if you were to think of a subluxation as a misalignment of a "cog" in the human spine, and an adjustment as putting that cog back into alignment, the analogy of body as machine still doesn't hold. Realigning a vertebra in the spine won't create the immediate effect that realigning a cog in a machine will, because of all the chemical and biological consequences of the misalignment. It takes time for the effect of the realignment to permeate the organism. Unlike fixing a machine, healing a human body is a process. *True healing takes time.*

Unfortunately, a lot of conventional medicine still operates from a largely unconscious mind-set of "fixing" the body rather than healing it. Most disease or illness is regarded as something that happens to us, rather than something caused or exacerbated by our lifestyle choices. Doctors use drugs and surgery to "fix" symptoms, and less frequently to address the causes of illness. However, quick fixes are rarely what the body truly needs to heal itself. In truth, every disease or injury is also a process, not an event. Cancer is a process. Heart disease is a process. A heart attack is a process, a cascade of biological events within the human body. Even a traumatic injury such as breaking an arm is not an isolated occurrence but a triggering impulse that causes changes to tissue, blood, lymph, hormones, and so on, not just at the site of the break but throughout the body. And in the same way that all injury or illness is a process, healing, too, is a series of positive changes over time that are designed to restore the body to its proper level of function.

I described in Chapter 4 how a skinned knee scabs and then grows new skin to cover the damaged area. In order for the body to heal properly, it needs time for the cells to organize and replace damaged tissue with tissue that's of the same quality. If the body has to replace cells quickly, the replacements are often less refined, bigger, less organized. A scab is a perfect example of this phenomenon. The skin cells that are part of the scab on a skinned knee are thicker, stiffer, and less refined, and they're laid down in clumps rather than in neat, tidy rows. The color doesn't match the skin surrounding the scab, and the cells don't function as well as the skin they're replacing. But the cells get into place quickly, to prevent infectious agents from entering the break in the skin. Innate Intelligence knows it needs to slap a patch on a breach in the body's defenses, and it is less concerned with looks and function than it is with filling the hole. To get real healing, however, you need time for new, organized skin cells to form beneath the scab. It can take a couple of weeks before the scab is completely replaced by pink, healthy cells, and a few weeks after that before the appearance and function of the knee is back to normal. True healing—defined as restoration of normal function—takes time because it is a process, not an event.

Maintaining your body's overall health is also a process—the process of a lifetime. If your health is affected adversely by injury, disease, aging, environmental, genetic and other factors, the process of restoring health will undoubtedly take time. In Western society, and especially in conventional Western medicine, we've been conditioned to believe in the quick fix. But to restore health at the deepest level, we must focus on healing the body instead of fixing it. This approach, which is advocated by chiropractic and alternative healing techniques, means that the healing process may take more time than popping a pill. But because the body is repairing itself at the deepest possible level, the health you gain will potentially last longer and be far more like the original state of health you were meant to have. This does not necessarily mean that a medical quick fix is without value, but we have to look carefully at the choices we make. Oftentimes short-term fixes may interfere with long-term healing.

Healing can be a process that causes positive, powerful transformation in our lives. Many people who have gone through serious illness or even faced death say that their lives are changed forever by the experience. If we choose to look at illness and healing as gifts, it changes the entire lens through which we view medicine and disease. If we are willing to learn from the process, the struggle for life and health has a universe of knowledge to teach us—even if the lesson learned is one of the most simple yet powerful: the appreciation of life.

▶ The Process of Ongoing Chiropractic Care

As I said in Chapter 7, on either your first or second visit with your chiropractor, he or she will probably recommend a course of treatment that includes a series of visits over a period of weeks or months. It's important that you are very clear about what to expect from your course of treatment. Although many patients do experience relief right away, chiropractic care is about healing rather than a "quick fix," and thus your symptoms may not disappear after your first visit, or even your third or fourth.

Going to a chiropractor is not like going to the medical doctor, where the problem gets cut out or disguised by drugs. Your body is being restored to healthy functioning, and that's a process in which there are many stages. After one adjustment, you might feel great; after the next, you may be sore. One day you may feel happy, and then a day later you're depressed for no reason. Everything from euphoria to pain, more or less mobility, may show up during your course of treatment. If you're worried about any symptoms or reactions, please make sure to talk to your chiropractor. But you should also realize that whatever you're experiencing is likely part of the process of your body restoring itself to full and natural function.

In truth, sometimes the aches and pains you experience as part of your recovery are very good signs—they indicate that those parts of the body are finally coming alive again, so to speak. Remember, chiropractic care deals with the central and peripheral nervous systems, which affect the most fundamental functioning of the human body on every possible level. When a nerve is damaged severely enough to the point that it's near death, it no longer has any feeling. There's no pain, no sensation of pins and needles—just numbness. We see this all the time with burn victims; the areas that are severely burned often have no sensation at all. But when nerves repair themselves, people experience certain sensations in a very predictable procession. First (unfortunately) is pain, then tingling, itching, sensitivity, and finally a gradual return to what we can call normal sensation. Your nerves may or may not be badly damaged enough by subluxation for you to go through all those stages of sensation during the healing process. But the nerves are connected with various parts and organs of the body, and those parts and organs may experience similar sensations as part of the healing cycle.

Many patients choose chiropractic care because they like its focus on healing rather than the "quick fix" of conventional medicine. But with the additional benefits of deep healing comes a responsibility for the patient to understand that healing takes time and to be willing to let the body go through its own natural healing process, even if that involves some discomfort along the way. Your chiropractor, too, has additional responsibilities: to educate you about the process of chiropractic care and to support the body's restoration of function in every way possible. This may include lifestyle counseling or taking the time to listen to your questions and concerns and answer them with compassion and understanding care.

Remember, chiropractic care is designed not just to restore function when the body is out of whack, but also to support your body's ongoing health by catching potential problems before they become serious. After your initial round of adjustments, your chiropractor may recommend some amount of maintenance care. Depending on the technique and philosophy of your chiropractor, these visits may range from once a week to once a month or less. I ask my patients to use their maintenance appointments as a way of keeping themselves on track with a healthy lifestyle.

When you enter chiropractic care, you are beginning a new relationship with your body, one where you are asked to take responsibility for your own health. Your chiropractor and other health care providers are there to support the lifestyle and health care choices you make. There is a well-known saying: "If it is to be, it is up to me." Your health is your responsibility, and with a few simple changes and choices, you can ensure that your life is a process of health and vibrancy instead of one of disease and decline.

▶ A Simple Prescription for a Healthy Life

In the last few chapters we've discussed the "chiropractic lifestyle," meaning the kinds of health and lifestyle choices that you can make to increase your level of health. When you make positive diet, exercise, and health care choices on a consistent basis, it's logical to expect that good health will be yours. But if you were to go to the gym once and then never exercise again, would you be in shape? If you eat healthfully one day a month and chow down on McDonald's, pork rinds, and Big Gulp sodas from 7-Eleven the rest of the time, what do you think your arteries and colon would look like? If you meditate or get a massage only when you're feeling completely stressed and do nothing the rest of the time, even though you're feeling anxious about your job or your relationship or your life in general, what will that do to your blood pressure or digestion? And certainly if you go to your chiropractor only when you throw your back out and stop going once the pain is gone, how effective do you think your chiropractic care will be in helping you stay healthy (as opposed to "fixing" your pain)?

All the choices I've talked about as part of the chiropractic lifestyle are just that: a *lifestyle,* meaning that you adopt them as part of your everyday life. If you do so, then I guarantee that over the long term you'll be adding more life to your life and more health to your ongoing experience of living. But remember what I said earlier: The best way to ensure your success in adopting the chiropractic lifestyle is to take baby steps. If you read this book and then go out and completely change your diet, start running five miles a day, meditate for an hour each morning and evening, and go to the chiropractor three times a week, I'm afraid you'll be setting yourself up for failure. I'd much rather you ease your way into a new exercise program by taking a walk three times a week, for example, the first month. Then continue to walk while you add more fresh fruits, vegetables, and grains to your diet in month 2 or 3. By month 4, 5, or 6 you may want to use some of the stress-reduction ideas, such as massage, or meditating five minutes a day. And throughout you should follow the treatment plan you and your chiropractor agree upon. By easing into your new lifestyle you stand a far greater chance of sticking to the changes you've made.

While you do so, however, remember that, just as with going to the gym, you can't expect the results of your health regimen to show up immediately. Progress is cumulative. Your health may not seem all that much better after a month of eating well, but take a look at how you feel three months, six months, one year down the line. A month after you begin a regular walking program, you'll probably see an increase in your energy and stamina. Meditate regularly and your stress level usually will go down. And of course, with regular adjustments you'll definitely notice a difference in your body's level of function. All of these small changes will add up to a very different, healthier life.

Contrary to what a lot of the media and conventional medicine would have us believe, health is not a complicated thing. You don't have to be a rocket scientist to figure out how to get and stay healthy. But I would like to propose a radical notion: I believe health is not something you find by either pursuing it in an all-out fashion or neglecting it completely. If you look at the overall health of a high-performance athlete and a couch potato, you might be surprised to discover that neither end of the spectrum is particularly good in the long run. Many high-performance athletes put such overwhelming stress on their bodies over such long periods of time that their health suffers as they grow older. And we all know the results of lack of exercise and lousy nutrition, as demonstrated by the couch potato! Health, in truth, is a golden mean. Do we need to do a lot of running and heavy-duty exercise? Do we need to shoot for the exact perfect body weight for our height and age? Probably not. The ultimate recipe for health is simple: Find the balance of activity, food, mental and physical rest, and supportive health care that will enable us to maintain vitality and energy no matter what our age or circumstance. For most of us, that means eating a balanced diet, taking a walk now and then, and getting regular chiropractic care. That simple recipe is what chiropractors refer to as health *assurance,* instead of health insurance, because it gives us the assurance we are doing the best we can to stay healthy.

There's only one caveat: There will always be cases where people do everything they can to stay healthy, yet still come down with a serious disease. That's life. No matter how much we do, there will be forces that are working against us as we try to maintain our health. I used to say to my patients, tongue in cheek, "You know, if you get really healthy and do everything just right, you'll never die." Of course, we all know that's not true. But the chiropractic lifestyle is like stacking the deck in our favor. If you want to stack the odds against you, drink a fifth of vodka and smoke two packs of cigarettes a day, and sit around watching television. Then you can be fairly well assured that you will die young and miserable. On the other hand, if you invest in health assurance by exercising a little on a regular basis, eating a fairly balanced diet, going to a chiropractor on a regular basis, and paying moderate attention to your health, you will most likely live longer and feel better. Find that golden mean of health for yourself by doing what you can to stack the deck in your favor. If you use baby steps, then I believe your success—and your health—will be assured.

12

Chiropractic for Children

A few months ago a patient named Debbie brought her six-week-old son, Reid, to my clinic. I had taken care of Debbie a few years earlier, but she had drifted away from chiropractic care—it just didn't fit into her busy lifestyle, she said. Then Debbie got pregnant with Reid. Unfortunately, it was a difficult labor and birth, and from the outset Reid had many health problems. By the time Debbie brought Reid to my clinic, the baby already had undergone five courses of antibiotics for various infections. He had trouble digesting breast milk, and seemed grumpy and unhappy all the time. Debbie's family finally convinced her to bring Reid to see me. After all, I was already taking care of three generations of their family, they said, and what harm could it do?

Reid's story was very similar to the story of Sarah I told you in the Introduction. I performed one small adjustment to the baby's neck, and Reid's health problems disappeared. Within a day he was able to digest Debbie's milk. His entire demeanor changed; he became a happy, calm baby, a joy to be around.

One of the greatest joys of being a chiropractor is in treating children, because they usually respond so quickly to care. Children's bones are malleable, constantly in transition, and that makes them heal much more quickly. This also means that children are in need of regular chiropractic care to make sure they grow up healthy. Chiropractic can help your children overcome the effects of the bumps and bruises common to childhood; it can support their healthy participation in sports and other activities; it can strengthen the immune system and improve concentration; and, as Reid's case proved, it can help with conditions such as breastfeeding difficulties and colic. Most important, chiropractic care helps support children's health naturally, eliminating the need for many drugs, antibiotics, surgeries, and other medical treatments that can produce unwanted and long-term side effects. I hope the next few pages will show you the value of chiropractic in giving your children the gift of health—a gift that can last a lifetime.

▶ Subluxation at Birth: An Unrecognized Epidemic

In 1986 a study was published based on research performed by a doctor of physical medicine, Dr. G. Gutmann, while he was working at a pediatric hospital in Germany. Germany has had government-sponsored health care longer than any other country, and its medical system is excellent. What's more, the medical community there recognizes the benefits of alternative medicine. (B. J. Palmer had brought chiropractic to Eastern Europe in the first part of the twentieth century, where it was widely accepted and adopted into the medical community. Indeed, many alternative medical professionals work side by side with conventional medical doctors in hospitals and clinical settings.) Dr. Gutmann studied approximately two thousand newborns and infants at this particular hospital, which was a top-rated modern pediatric facility. Of the two thousand newborns, 221 had significant health problems in the first few days of life. In this population of 221 "unhealthy" infants, Dr. Gutmann found the incidence of subluxation to be 95 percent. Correction of these subluxations generated dramatic improvement in the health of nearly all the infants treated. Dr. Gutmann also found that approximately 75 percent of the two thousand children he examined had "atlas blockage," or subluxation of the top neck bone. So although the incidence of subluxation was even more prevalent in infants with health problems, 75 percent of the total population of children were having their potential for life diminished due to subluxation—and these were births with top-notch medical care! Dr. Gutmann recommended that chiropractors be present at all births, especially difficult ones, so they could check the children shortly after they're born for any problems.

Another study done in the United States implicates subluxation in sudden infant death syndrome (SIDS) and stillbirths. In 1968 Abraham Towbin, M.D., of the Boston University Medical Center, did autopsies on children who had died of SIDS or were stillborn, and found that on average seven out of eight had damage in the upper neck/brain stem area. Since then, additional studies delving into the causes of SIDS have indicated cervical instability in the brain stem area.

It is clear from these studies that many children are afflicted with problems with the neck and spine from the moment they're born. How could this be? There are several factors that create such trauma. First, the mother's own spinal and nerve health will have an enormous effect on her pregnancy and labor. If subluxation and structural imbalances occur in a pregnant woman and she is not under chiropractic care, probably her hips are tilted and twisted a little bit. Carrying a child puts enormous strain on a woman's body. Not only is she carrying anywhere from fifteen to forty pounds of extra weight, but most of that weight is in front of her. To compensate for the load, women end up walking, sitting, lying, and moving differently, all of which can put undue stress on the spine. In addition, the expanded uterus is pushing against many internal organs, causing even more physiological stress. Most pregnant women experience interference with the function of nerves as well as impingement on the structural and muscular systems.

Without regular chiropractic care during pregnancy, when a woman goes into labor her whole system isn't working as smoothly as it could. Her hips may be out of alignment; her spine itself may be torqued in subtle ways, enough to interfere with the birth process. When the baby tries to move down the birth canal, instead of gliding down smoothly it has to twist and turn to get out, creating more trauma for the child and a longer labor for the mother. However, when a woman has undergone regular chiropractic care during her pregnancy, the birthing process is usually smoother and easier, the way nature intends it to be. It's also often shorter. Some studies indicate that the labor of women under chiropractic care during pregnancy is 60 percent shorter than that of women who haven't had such care.

Even with a short, uneventful labor, however, babies are still at risk for subluxation. Most births in Western societies occur in hospitals with doctors present. It is not my objective to be negative about medical doctors, as they are simply doing what they were taught, but what they're taught can create problems for the baby. During the birth, when the baby's head appears the doctor typically uses the head to turn the baby's body—basically using the head as a lever to pull the baby out. This puts a lot of pressure on the baby's neck. I have read that in a normal birth a child experiences approximately eighty linear pounds of pressure on its neck. (Imagine someone pulling on your neck using about eighty pounds of force.) And that's in a normal birth. If there are problems, doctors use forceps, suction cups, and other devices to extract the child. I'm not saying such measures aren't necessary at times, but they certainly can cause great trauma to the child's neck and spine.

Plus, when a baby's born, most of its bones aren't even bone! A newborn child's skeletal structure is mostly cartilage, very soft and pliable. In some ways this is good, as it makes it possible for the baby to squeeze through the birth canal without breaking anything. But these tissues are also far more susceptible to trauma created by intervention. With all these factors, it's no wonder that Dr. Gutmann's study found that 75 percent of newborns suffered from some degree of misalignment and impingement in the upper neck.

Luckily, since children's bones are so malleable, and since babies heal extremely quickly, correcting an infant's subluxation is easy. I usually request that my patients bring their babies to see me within the first week—the sooner the better. Often I find that if the mother has had regular chiropractic care during her pregnancy, the baby has no subluxations at all, or perhaps a small amount of tension in the neck that can be relieved by a gentle light-force adjustment. (As you read in the Introduction, a light-force adjustment applies an extremely small amount of pressure on a trigger point to ease the bone back into place. Often holding a few ounces of pressure on the joint for thirty seconds will allow the muscles and bone to realign themselves.)

If a baby's subluxations go uncorrected, however, the results may not be clearly linked to misalignment of the spine. As you saw in the examples of Reid and Sarah, uncorrected subluxations can create digestive problems, impede normal growth, and cause a child to develop allergies. Subluxations also can cause constipation. I had one young patient whom I first saw when he was about eight months old. His mother brought him from Olympia, a city about three hours away from my clinic. This little boy had severe torticollis, meaning his head was tilted almost completely to one side. I told the mother, "Typically with this kind of subluxation there are digestive problems; either the baby won't keep food down or has constipation." The mother admitted that her son had extreme constipation; since the first week after his birth they had to give him a suppository every day because he couldn't have a bowel movement. (I've seen this symptom a number of times, not only in babies but with adults and older kids as well. When you interfere with the nervous system in the upper neck or in the lower back, it can greatly affect the body's ability to eliminate properly.) I checked the child, found a subluxation in the upper neck, adjusted the baby—and the next day the baby pooped so much, they could hardly keep him in diapers! Constipation was never a problem again for this child.

A well-known saying in chiropractic is "As the twig is bent, so grows the tree." In the same way that it's far easier to bend a twig than a full-grown tree trunk, it's easier to make small adjustments to children's bones and joints that will heal subluxations and help children grow in the way Innate Intelligence meant them to. But as always, the sooner the subluxation is addressed, the sooner healing can begin.

▶ Healing the Bumps and Bruises of Childhood

When I was four years old, my family lived in Indiana. Our next-door neighbors were the Hipskins, an older couple we called Grandma and Grandpa because they were so nice. The Hipskins had a big backyard, and in it was an old-fashioned clothesline. It consisted of a single four-by-four post topped by two four-by-fours shaped like an X, with a clothesline draped between the arms of the X. The whole thing must have weighed more than a hundred pounds.

One winter day I was playing in the Hipskins' backyard. I was wearing a red coat with a fake white fleece lining and a hood. The wind was blowing especially hard, and all of a sudden it blew over the clothesline. Bam! The four-by-four post landed right on top of my head. It felt like I was a nail being driven into the ground. I lay there dazed for a few minutes, then I picked myself up, put my hood over my head, and ran home. When I saw my mom, I started crying. She pushed my hood back and almost went into shock because it was full of blood. She rushed me to the hospital, and I had to have a number of stitches in my scalp.

No one thought there would be any aftereffects of the accident, but when I was six or seven I started suffering from severe "growing pains"—intense aches and pains that would move from one spot to another. My parents took me to an orthopedist and a neurologist, but neither could find anything wrong with me. Eventually I grew out of my growing pains, but when I got into junior high school I started having really severe migraine headaches. I wouldn't be able to move for seventy-two hours: I'd have to lie in a dark room with a towel over my eyes, perfectly still. If I moved my head even a quarter of an inch, it felt like there was somebody inside my head with an ax trying to get out. I'd throw up for hours. It was awful.

Luckily, I eventually grew out of the migraines, too, but then in my late teens and early twenties, I suffered from chronic neck and back pain. You would think at some point I might have tried chiropractic, right? But my parents didn't believe in it, so it wasn't until I injured a shoulder when I was twenty-five that I finally went to see a chiropractor. As I told you in the Introduction, at that visit I decided this was the profession for me.

In chiropractic school I had my first set of really comprehensive X rays, and I finally discovered the reason for all my aches and pains growing up. When that clothesline post had fallen on my head, it had split my atlas bone—the bone at the very top of the neck, where it joins to the skull—in half. It's what's called a decompression or Jackson fracture. You see it in people who are in diving accidents, where they jump headfirst into shallow water and hit their heads. The fracture had literally split my atlas bone into two pieces. That injury probably caused my very first subluxation; it was at the root of all the aches and pains I had had growing up, all the migraines, and all the neck and back pain.

From a chiropractic point of view, the concept of "growing pains" is fictitious. The normal process of growing shouldn't hurt. We talked a little in Chapter 5 about the cumulative effect of abnormal range of motion on the joints of the body and the spine. The same cumulative effect holds true in early life. The lumps and bumps of childhood can create subluxations that begin to take their toll on the health of the spine and joints. If left untreated, these subluxations can cause the kinds of problems I experienced. When I finally sought treatment, because my injury had been left alone for over twenty years it took quite a while—about seven years—to get my spine back to optimal health. That's one of the reasons I am such an advocate of regular chiropractic care for children.

Every child is going to experience some bumps and bruises as he or she grows. Babies fall off changing tables. Toddlers tumble off tricycles or out of cribs. Kids get banged up in many ways—bicycles, tree houses, skating, running, all kinds of sports—in the normal process of growing up. For the most part, children's bodies are growing and regenerating at such a rapid pace that minor injuries like these aren't a problem. However, sometimes the damage is severe enough to cause problems later; in other cases, the cumulative effect of minor traumas can create long-term challenges. Luckily, chiropractic is uniquely suited to address many of the injuries of even the most active child.

In the same way that good food and regular exercise are important in helping a child's body to develop healthfully, regular chiropractic care can train a child's bones, joints, nerves, and muscles to function at optimal efficiency. Luckily, children don't need a lot of care. It's not like an adult who comes in at sixty-five years of age with cumulative damage from years of trauma. Unless there has been some sort of trauma or congenital condition, I usually see children who are patients about once every three months. Regular adjustments not only eliminate any consequences of the usual bumps and bruises of childhood, but they also create a pattern of health that children's bodies can follow for the rest of their lives.

Of course, there still are times when a child is injured and the parents should take the child to a conventional medical doctor— if the child has fallen and broken a bone, for example, or has an injury that breaks the skin. Certainly I am very grateful that when

I got hit in the head and lacerated my scalp at age four, my mother took me to the hospital to get my head stitched up! But if there has been a fall or other kind of accident, in many cases I suggest parents also take their child to see the chiropractor as soon as possible to make sure that any subluxations are found and healed. Of course, if the family is following a regular regimen of chiropractic care (four or more visits per year), there's usually no reason to bring the child in for a special visit unless there is a significant trauma; the regularly scheduled visit will usually catch anything that has occurred in the last few weeks. At such routine visits I ask both the child and the parents if there have been any falls or injuries since the last time I saw the child, but in truth, my usual patient assessment will pick up most subluxations that have appeared.

Bringing your child to see a chiropractor following an injury or fall can be very beneficial and will certainly do no harm. Chiropractors are trained in diagnosis and assessment, and they will not hesitate to refer a child to a medical doctor if they believe it's necessary. (Unfortunately, the reverse is not true: Few conventional doctors will refer a child to a chiropractor for treatment of injury or trauma even when such treatment might be clearly indicated, as in the case of whiplash or strain on the spine. Conventional doctors are more likely to prescribe a drug than to look to alternative means of healing the body.) For example, chiropractors all recognize the symptoms and signs of a concussion, one of the more serious consequences of a childhood fall. Concussion obviously requires specific diagnosis, treatment, and follow-up, and certain aspects of the appropriate treatment for severe concussion fall within the conventional medical model. However, I do recommend that children who have suffered a concussion come to see me within a week so that I can check the neck and spine for subluxations that probably have occurred. (If a child has hit his or her head hard enough to cause a concussion, chances are there's been enough stress on the spine and joints to produce subluxations.)

All parents feel the responsibility of making important decisions for their children—about their health, education, habits, and other lifestyle issues. I believe that chiropractic care can be a very powerful tool to help parents bring up healthy, happy, vital children. It is also my belief that adopting chiropractic care as a regular part of a family's health care regimen can provide enormous benefit as well as great peace of mind for all concerned. Furthermore, it teaches kids that their body can heal itself from within and that they don't need drugs to treat every ache and pain.

▶ Chiropractic and Childhood Sports

Nowhere is there a greater need for consistent chiropractic support than with children who play sports. Whether they're involved in peewee and Pop Warner football, Little League baseball, weekend soccer games, or gymnastics, the amount of stress and strain placed on our children's growing bodies—on bones and joints that are still forming—is enormous. The danger of injury from either trauma or repetitive abnormal motion is also increased.

If you have any doubts about the need for additional physical support for children who engage in sports, look at the people who make sports their life: professional athletes (and I include Olympic athletes in that category). We admire these individuals because they push their bodies to the limit. However, the toll this takes is beyond the body's capacity to repair in the normal course of events. Professional athletes are often some of the unhealthiest people around. What's more unfortunate, in many sports the peak physical age for that activity is anywhere from the preteen years to the early twenties. These young people we so admire for their physical achievements are causing horrendous damage to their bones, muscles, and joints because of the huge demands placed on them by their sports.

It's no surprise to me that so many of these professional athletes rely on drugs and sports medicine specialists to get them past their pain. If you want to achieve exceptional performance over the long term, however, drugs and surgical intervention can only do so much (and can even cause more damage than they cure). Nutritional supplements, massage, and especially chiropractic care form an important part of the health care regimen of many professional athletes. And I believe that anyone else who plays sports regularly should make chiropractic care a part of their regular routine.

Of course, the schedule of treatments will depend on the kind of sport being played and the child's level of activity. If your child is involved in a contact sport, such as football, I recommend he be checked once a week during the season. For sports such as soccer, basketball, baseball, volleyball, or tennis, bringing the child in every other week or once a month usually is sufficient. Obviously, if the child suffers any kind of injury in the course of the sport, I suggest the parent bring the child in as soon as possible.

Let me say a special word about gymnastics. This sport is very tough on the body, not just because of the athletic demands but also because of the flexibility required. The tender age of the children involved (especially for girls) means that the bones and joints are still forming, and the range of motion required by many gymnastic moves is certainly far greater than normal. This puts a lot of stress on the joints and can create both subluxations and other damage to the soft tissues. I've heard of children in their teens receiving regular cortisone shots to help them overcome the pain in their joints so they can keep competing! I regard this as intolerable. A combination of regular chiropractic care and a sane approach to competing and training will allow these children to enjoy sports while making sure their bodies will be healthy long after they stop competing.

One final point about chiropractic and sports: There have been a number of studies that suggest chiropractic can enhance athletic ability and performance by as much as 18 percent. Athletes who receive regular chiropractic care find it helps keep their structure strong, aids proprioception (spatial and muscular perception), and promotes proper muscle and nervous system balance—in general, they perform at a higher level. It also can help protect against some of the damage that competitive sports can inflict on the body.

▶ Chiropractic and Scoliosis

Scoliosis, or curvature of the spine, is usually first detected during childhood. The condition is divided into several different categories. Frequently doctors can't determine the cause of the curvature; that kind of scoliosis is called *idiopathic* (the diagnosis in upward of 70 percent of cases). In other cases, the scoliosis is caused by malformation of a vertebra during the development of the child before birth. This kind of structural scoliosis is *congenital.*

Scoliosis is measured by the degree of lateral (side-to-side) curvature from the normally straight line of the backbone. Mild scoliosis would be under 15 degrees, moderate up to 25 degrees, and severe over 35 degrees. If not corrected, scoliosis in children and teenagers usually will progress to ever greater degrees of curvature. Extreme scoliosis can crush the lungs, inhibit the person's ability to breathe, and affect other organs. Even a mild case of scoliosis produces problems in the back, hips, knees, and feet, due to the fact that one side of the body is higher than the other.

Treatment options offered by conventional medicine range from braces, casts, and exercises to corrective surgery. Unfortunately, these options are frequently painful and embarrassing for the child, and can result in time away from school and normal childhood activities. Since scoliosis involves the spine, patients whose children have the condition will often ask their chiropractors if there are any natural alternatives. And there is evidence that chiropractic care and other forms of alternative medicine can be helpful in some types of scoliosis.

Chiropractors don't necessarily perform scoliosis screenings of their patients, although some do. But they *do* perform postural analysis, and that often will pick up any abnormal curvature of the spine. When a child comes into our clinic for the first time we always do a postural analysis, and occasionally follow up with X rays. (Most chiropractors will not X-ray children unless they feel it's absolutely necessary.) If there is any indication of abnormalities in the spine, we will do a thorough workup and usually prescribe a series of adjustments to bring the bones and soft tissues in the joints back to healthful function.

Many chiropractors who specialize in scoliosis maintain that what medical doctors call idiopathic scoliosis is oftentimes really the result of structural and neurological imbalances caused by subluxations that are throwing the spine out of balance and creating abnormal curvature. That's why chiropractic care alone will resolve some cases, especially if the condition is mild and not congenital (that is, not produced by problems in bone formation). Chiropractic can also slow down or stop the process of spinal curvature by strengthening the supporting nerves and joints. If the scoliosis continues to develop, or if it is severe when the child is brought in, then chiropractors have been known to work in conjunction with orthopedists to correct the problem. A combination of body casts, exercises, and regular chiropractic care (again, to support the restoration of normal joint and spinal functioning) has been shown to be beneficial in many cases.

With severe scoliosis, the cause may originate in the brain or in the formation of bones before birth. In such cases medical intervention may be necessary. However, since one of the stated aims of regular chiropractic care is to improve muscle and nerve function and to return the body to optimal condition, it is almost always beneficial to continue to receive adjustments even if medical treatment is needed. This is especially true given the fact that most medical doctors will not intervene surgically until the scoliosis reaches approximately a 40 percent curvature. So if your child has anything less than that, chiropractic care may be one of your first resorts. Depending on the child, chiropractic may be able to resolve the condition completely. It certainly can aid in the restoration of the spine to normal function.

▶ Chiropractic and Childhood Illness

Far too many parents end up taking their children to the doctor constantly to treat this illness, that infection, or some other unspecified ailment. They spend hours in waiting rooms and cough up far too much money for doctor visits and prescriptions to treat symptoms, only to have the illness recur a few weeks later. But as I hope I've demonstrated throughout this book, there is another choice parents can make when it comes to the health of their children—one that promotes health rather than treating symptoms, and has the additional benefit of teaching children a healthier approach to their own bodies.

You wouldn't necessarily think that chiropractic could help children overcome physical ailments such as allergies, digestive problems, ear infections, and chronic tonsillitis. But I've seen all of these conditions improved or even eliminated with regular chiropractic care. For example, in a 1988 study done with 217 children treated at Western States Chiropractic College, substantial improvement was seen in 61.6 percent of children with complaints such as ear infections, sinus problems, allergies, bedwetting, or respiratory and gastrointestinal problems, with 60.6 percent seeing "maximum" improvement. (See Appendix I for more information on many of these conditions.) Reid, the baby whom you met at the beginning of this chapter, had had five courses of antibiotics by the time he was six weeks old, and yet he became a healthy, happy baby with just a few adjustments.

Studies of the effects of regular chiropractic care on ailments such as allergies and infections are ongoing. But researchers theorize that there is a correlation between adjustment of the spine and improvement in the immune system. On a direct level, after an adjustment we can see distinct changes in chemical levels that are directly related to the pituitary and thyroid glands, both of which affect the immune system. But the real effect goes back to the fundamental principles of chiropractic that we discussed in Chapter 5. We know that if we sever a nerve that goes to an organ in the body, that organ will begin to die. Therefore, the health of any tissue in the body is affected by the health of the nerve that is connected to it. Subluxations cause interference with proper firing of the nerves that extend from the spinal cord to all the organs and limbs of the body. For instance, if the nerves that go to the nasal passages, throat, or the bronchi in the lungs become unhealthy as a result of subluxation, then over time the tissues those nerves go to also will become unhealthy. And when these tissues become unhealthy, they become more susceptible to irritants, infection, and disease. The body's response to these irritants then expresses itself as symptoms such as sinus infections, hay fever, other allergies, and chronic tonsillitis.

Conventional medicine will treat the symptoms (with pain relievers, antihistamines, cough medicine, and other drugs) or will try to treat the condition by eliminating the substances that are irritating the body or by desensitizing the body to the foreign substance. But it rarely looks at the underlying *cause* of the symptoms, which is the fundamental lack of health of the body. Chiropractic adjustments don't treat symptoms, but they do treat the body's real problem: interference with proper nerve functioning. When the nerves are restored to health, all the organs and limbs are receiving the proper kinds of instruction, which allows them to respond healthfully to irritants, foreign substances, bacteria, and so on. The result? Fewer trips to the doctor, fewer medications, increased health for the child—and greater peace of mind for parents.

Let's take the case of ear infection, or otitis media. According to Tedd Koren, D.C. (editor of a comprehensive compendium of chiropractic and spinal research done over the last several years), by the age of three over two-thirds of all children in the United States have had at least one ear infection. Antibiotics are the prescription of choice for conventional medical doctors and parents alike. But what if chiropractic could provide a viable alternative to antibiotics—indeed, what if it could prevent ear infections in the first place? In one seminal study in 1989 comparing the health of children of pediatricians with that of children of chiropractors, more than 80 percent of pediatricians' children suffered at least one instance of otitis media, compared to only 31 percent of chiropractors' children. A later study (1997) involved 332 children anywhere from twenty-seven days to five years of age, with otitis media that ranged from mild to severe, acute to chronic. All of the children in the study experienced some improvement in their conditions with chiropractic adjustments alone (no antibiotics). It took anywhere from five to six adjustments for the condition to normalize itself over a period of seven to eleven days. And the recurrence rate was as low as 11 percent when tracked over a six-month period.

Of course, I'm not saying parents should never take their children to the doctor when illness occurs. Just as with trauma, some illnesses need the kind of immediate intervention provided by the drugs and surgery of conventional medicine. However, many childhood ailments tend to be chronic (recurring) rather than acute, and it is those ailments where the ongoing health support of chiropractic care can provide a safe, sane alternative. My own daughter, who is now twenty-one, received regular chiropractic care from birth, and I can remember giving her antibiotics only twice in her entire life (unlike her friends, who seemed to be on all kinds of medication throughout childhood).

It is important for parents to remember that while the results of chiropractic care are ultimately healthier for the child, the actual treatment of the condition may take some time. When a chiropractor corrects a subluxation, it's like fertilizing the roots of a tree: The effects of that fertilizer travel gradually from the roots through the trunk to the branches and leaves. Even though the impact may not be apparent right away, ultimately the entire tree will be far healthier for the fertilizer. In the same way, when a subluxation is corrected, it takes time for the nerves and soft tissues around the spine to heal and start sending the correct signals to the target tissue. Once that happens, it also will take time for the target tissue itself to heal and start responding correctly to the environment.

I always caution my patients—children, parents, or otherwise— not to expect instant results when it comes to treating illnesses such as chronic infection or allergies. I remind people that chiropractic is about treating causes, not symptoms. I tell them that the health of their bodies will increase as soon as proper functioning of nerves is restored, and then the rest of the body will experience healing and restoration of function as well.

▶ Raising Healthier Children Without Drugs

We've all heard about the consequences of the overprescription of antibiotics: how conventional medical doctors used to prescribe antibiotics at the drop of a hat, only to realize that bacteria were becoming resistant to the medications that are supposed to kill them. Now even conventional doctors try to avoid overprescribing antibiotics, and parents are the ones demanding the drugs they see as a cure for every childhood illness. It would seem logical that parents would be delighted to find another, drug-free choice to keep their children healthy.

Chiropractic teaches children an approach to health and healing that is far different from and more wholesome than the traditional medical model. The medical model teaches us that when we're sick, we take a pill. Whenever a child feels ill, parents tell them, "Here, take Tylenol, take Dimetapp. It will make you feel better." Then when the kids become teenagers, their parents say, "Don't take drugs"—when they've been taking drugs their whole lives! We're teaching children that if you feel bad and want to feel good, you take something outside your body and put it into your body. Is it any wonder that children who have been raised on chewable Tylenol, Dimetapp lollipops, and cold medication that tastes like grape soda turn to illegal drugs as a way of feeling good? Or that they abuse steroids, diet pills, laxatives, tranquilizers, and other medications in their desire to be stronger, thinner, or happier?

There is a better way, one that promotes health and healing rather than disguising symptoms with "quick fix" medications, one that teaches children to work with their bodies rather than rely on drugs to feel good. Part of every parent's responsibility is deciding how his or her children should be raised, and that includes how they wish them to view health, healing, and medicine. Obviously, my bias is toward a more natural approach because I believe ultimately it will best serve the child's long-term health. The natural approach creates a completely different mindset, lifestyle, and psychology.

One of the most painful and confusing dilemmas faced by parents today has to do with using drugs to treat children's behavioral problems. We are giving powerful drugs to children as young as three, with almost no information about their long-term effects! For instance, Ritalin (commonly prescribed for hyperactivity) is a stimulant and can be addictive if abused; nowadays kids are selling it on the street and taking it inappropriately. Ritalin abuse also seems to be potentially associated with psychosis later in life. And let's take a look at the side effects even when Ritalin is used correctly: loss of appetite, stomach pain, weight loss, problems sleeping, and abnormal heart rhythm. Yet an entire generation of children is on Prozac, Ritalin, and other mood-altering medications because their desperate parents have been told that is the best solution for their children's behavioral problems. I'm not blaming parents or even the medical establishment, but I want to stand on the rooftops and shout, "There is another way!" I encourage my patients and their children to take a multipronged approach to dealing with childhood ailments, whether physical or behavioral. It's important to start by looking at the big picture, to examine every part of the child's life and health, from diet to spinal health to emotional issues to perceptual difficulties to physical challenges.

For instance, I have many patients who have been diagnosed with attention deficit hyperactivity disorder (ADHD), and there always seems to be a number of factors present. Treating any or all of these factors can result in an improvement in the condition without resorting to drugs. Sometimes there are subluxations present, and when the subluxations are treated the child becomes calmer and more focused. (A recent study done at a chiropractic college in Australia shows that chiropractic adjustments increase mental clarity. Personally, many of my patients, both children and adults, tell me that when they get adjusted, their thinking clears up.) In other cases, food allergies have been shown to play a role in ADHD, and changing a child's diet will dramatically change his behavior. In still other cases, the problem may be due to the way the child learns and thinks. As a society, we value a certain kind of thinking, the kind that does well with group-based education aimed at a middle level of intelligence. ADHD kids often just don't fit the mold. Either they can't learn using the ways information is traditionally presented in a classroom (and become enormously frustrated as a result), or the ways they express themselves don't jibe with classroom demands. Some children who are diagnosed with ADHD have later been shown to be extremely smart. Essentially they are acting out because they are bored silly by their environment. Others are overstimulated by their environment and need a more structured and calmer atmosphere. Either way, teachers who are struggling to satisfy the needs of the majority of students don't have either the time or the energy to take care of one child's individualized needs.

I don't want to oversimplify complex behavioral problems that many parents and children are struggling to deal with daily. I just want to suggest that drugs should be the *last* option rather than the first, especially when it comes to treating our children in the long run. In some cases, alternative health support can reduce or eliminate the need for drugs. But I believe *every* child can benefit from improving his or her health through diet, exercise, intellectual stimulation, and regular chiropractic care.

▶ The Immunization Controversy

One final word about a very controversial topic: childhood immunizations. Immunizations are something that every parent must deal with, as most schools require proof of immunization before they will allow a child to attend. Yet many parents who prefer to support their own and their children's health through more natural means are uncertain about the value of immunizations. And since chiropractors have been in the forefront of natural medicine in the United States for the past hundred years, immunization has been hotly debated in our ranks.

Both sides of the immunization issue have what they consider strong proofs of their positions. Pro-immunizers point to the near elimination of childhood illnesses such as polio, measles, mumps, diphtheria, and so on—diseases that were all too common in the early twentieth century. They say that immunization must be mandatory to control any potential outbreaks of these contagious diseases. They remind us that immunizations are almost homeopathic, since they use a small amount of germs to stimulate the body's own immune system, and therefore almost could be considered a nondrug intervention. According to these advocates, the downside of these immunizations is minimal when applied to the population as a whole.

Anti-immunizers counter that thousands of children each year have adverse reactions to immunizations, including convulsions, neurological damage, even death. They question the validity of "experimenting" on an entire population using biological substances for which we can only begin to guess the long-term effects. They argue that the increasing number of immunizations given to children may be responsible for the rise in the occurrence of autoimmune diseases in the United States. (Immunizations are designed to produce antibodies to disease. There is speculation, and some research that validates it, that immunizations also increase the amount of a very specific chemical known as gamma globulin in the body, and overproduction of gamma globulin is implicated in autoimmune diseases.)

Anti-immunizers also argue that, regardless of the effectiveness or ineffectiveness of immunization, the government has no right to make any kind of health treatment mandatory. (Actually, contrary to public belief, immunization is not mandatory. Almost all states allow for exemptions based on religious belief, and the state of Washington allows philosophic belief as a basis for exemption as well.) They question whether it's proper for the government to promote one form of health care and one healing philosophy, and make it difficult for people who don't conform.

As a parent, you are responsible for making choices when it comes to the health of your children. I have faced this challenge myself as a parent, and I see patients every day who wish to make the best choices for their children. Especially when it comes to immunizations, I tell patients, "Your most important job is to make an informed choice. If there were an immunization that had never shown an adverse response, was not required by the government, and I believed my children needed protection from that particular disease, certainly I would be willing to get them immunized. But there are adverse effects to many vaccines, and there also are consequences to buying into wholesale immunization without doing some investigation first. Look at all sides and make the decision you feel fits with what you want for your children and your own philosophy of health and well-being. Have an open mind. Be willing to think about the issue; don't just follow along with any philosophy, whether it's Christian Science or the scientific method. Your job as a parent is to get as much information as you can, and then make the decision that you feel is best for your child. And that includes keeping them as healthy as possible by strengthening the body through natural means such as chiropractic, diet, and exercise."

Robert S. Mendelsohn, M.D., author of *Confessions of a Medical Heretic,* states that parents are really the best assessors of their child's health and health care needs. There is no doctor in the world who knows your children better than you do—how they act when they're healthy, what happens when they're not feeling quite right, and the kind of care that will serve your children best. I believe chiropractic can serve as a powerful and helpful means to keep your children healthy naturally, with fewer sick days, less need for any kinds of medication, and a happier state of mind.

13

Chiropractic for Seniors

Recently I treated a very special person, Mildred, who was ninety-five years old. She was brought to my clinic by friends who were patients of mine. Mildred was a very funny lady and very sharp, but as you can imagine, at ninety-five she was a little frail physically. She told me she had a few aches and pains, along with some problems with dizziness and balance. But the thing that bothered her most was the fact that the top of her head was numb. "I want you to take this 'hat' off my head!" she told me.

We performed our usual series of diagnostic tests, took X rays, and then adjusted Mildred's upper neck. In our offices, after we do upper neck adjustments we have the patients lie down for a while and rest. Some even take a quick nap in the rooms we have set aside for that purpose. Well, when Mildred woke up from her postadjustment nap, she said, "Dr. Lenarz, it's the strangest thing: I can see!"

I thought, *That's interesting* —*she didn't say anything about a problem with her vision.* Then Mildred explained that fifteen years earlier she had fallen and hit her head. From that point on she had had double vision. One of the things she had loved her whole life was reading, but after the fall she couldn't read anymore. For fifteen years she had put up with the problem, but after one adjustment and a forty-minute rest, her double vision was gone.

Just think of what we consider the "inevitable" signs of aging: aches and pains in the joints, decreased mobility, lower energy, less acuity of both the senses and the mind, lowered resistance to disease. But are all these truly inevitable? Of course not. We all know individuals who stay healthy and vital well into their senior years. What makes them different? I believe it is due to their working to maintain their bodies at the highest level of function possible. These senior role models use diet, exercise, and good mental attitude to keep themselves young. And as I can testify from treating hundreds of senior citizens myself, many of them use chiropractic as a valuable part of their ongoing health care.

If you think the spine has little to do with health as we age, take a look at the people in their sixties, seventies, and eighties who are in nursing homes, and then look at people the same age who participate in activities at senior centers. You will notice very distinct and obvious differences in posture. The ones in nursing homes tend to be arthritic and bent over, and the ones at the senior centers are doing exercises and dancing; they have good, strong posture. If some of the stereotypes of aging are the bent back, the shrinking body, and the "dowager's hump" for both women and men, it should be obvious that it would be to our benefit to keep our spines as healthy as possible as we age. Indeed, there appears to be a strong correlation between quality and longevity of life and the health of the spine and nervous system.

But of course, chiropractic doesn't simply help the posture. In truth, chiropractic treats nerves, joints, and bones, helping them maintain optimal levels of function no matter what our age. Certainly, many seniors come to chiropractors because they have been experiencing pain, often for years. But what they find is an improvement in overall function that makes them feel more healthy and vital. I look at someone like Winifred, the lady I described in Chapter 1, who came to see me for chronic back pain and as a result of treatment was able to sleep through the night for the first time in years. Or Dan, the World War II veteran who saw his back pain and headaches vanish, and even stopped wearing the trifocal glasses he had used for fifty years. I have known senior citizens who are in better health than some of the thirty-year-olds who come to see me, simply because the senior citizens take better care of themselves and get regular chiropractic care.

▶ Degeneration May Be Inevitable, but It Is Treatable

One of the definitions of aging is the degeneration of physical and mental functioning. Certainly we all will degenerate until the forces of entropy eventually overtake us and we are no longer alive; our very cells seem to have a certain life span built into their DNA. However, there is a difference between the degeneration caused by entropy and our bodies' normal functioning over time, on one hand, and the excessive wear and tear as a result of bad habits and environmental stresses, on the other. This is the difference between *physical* and *chronological* age. There are some individuals who are eighty years old chronologically but possess the physical age and vitality of fifty-year-olds. And there are fifty-year-olds who look and feel eighty. The rate at which we age is determined to some degree by genetics, but for the most part it is determined by how we take care of ourselves at every stage of life.

Chiropractors see the beginning of degenerative changes in the spines of patients of all ages. I've seen many patients in their thirties and forties who come in complaining of a range of symptoms that are the result of long-standing untreated subluxations. As you learned in Chapter 5, subluxations cause inflammation and deterioration of the soft tissue supporting the bones of the spine. If left untreated, subluxations can cause the muscles, bones, and nerves to degenerate, leading to osteoarthritis, thinning of disks, formation of bone spurs, muscle weakness, nerve interference that can cause numbness and lack of function (like Mildred, the lady I described at the beginning of this chapter). If left untreated, these changes become more and more accentuated as the years go by. Natural degeneration coupled with subluxation accelerates the aging process.

Because the effects of degeneration are cumulative and usually take a long time to appear (and especially because many people have bought into the idea that aging equals degeneration), far too many seniors accept their limited mobility and aches and pains as a fact of life rather than something that can be helped. They accept that they can't reach as high or carry as much anymore; they believe it's normal for their senses to dim and their joints to be stiff. They say, "Oh well, this is what getting old is all about." But there's a significant difference between getting old and getting old with subluxations; getting old with subluxations is a much more unpleasant experience. Luckily, sometimes the smallest amount of care will make a major difference in how seniors feel.

Seniors' bones are all too often "frozen" by years of abnormal motion and lack of proper chiropractic maintenance. They need regular care to help unlock the joints and repair the damage that has occurred over time. By maintaining the health of the spine and nervous system, chiropractic care can help mitigate or eliminate many of the complaints we associate with aging. Whenever you correct subluxation, you reduce the extra stress and strain the joints are under. This increases mobility and energy levels, decreases pain, and improves nerve function. Regular chiropractic care can aid us not only when we are young and growing but also when we are older, helping us have healthier spines and nervous systems and stronger structure. And for many active seniors in their sixties and seventies, regular chiropractic care allows them to exercise and retain their mobility and energy levels.

It is important to note, however, that the older you get, the longer your course of chiropractic treatment may need to be. Let's go back to the tree metaphor I used when talking about children and chiropractic. Imagine your spine as a tree. It's growing straight and strong, and then all of a sudden, something happens to kink the trunk in one direction or another. The tree adapts and starts growing crooked. The longer the tree is allowed to grow crooked, the more bent over and gnarled it becomes. The same thing happens with the human body. If you've had a subluxation in place for a long time, your body has adapted to it. The longer a subluxation is in place, the more permanent the damage to the local tissue, and the more adapted the body becomes to a lesser degree of functioning.

One of the ways in which chiropractors assess a patient's condition is by evaluating how much degeneration shows up on an X ray. Degeneration is divided into three phases. In phase one, typically the neck or a part of the spine has lost its normal biomechanical positioning. For example, when you look at an X ray of the neck from the side view, it should have a gentle, forward-sloping curve. A loss in the curvature of the neck would be considered phase one of subluxation degeneration. When you lose the curvature of the neck, it causes extra wear and tear on the joints of the neck and spine, and that accelerates the degenerative processes.

In phase two you begin to see thinning of the disks and formation of bone spurs. In phase three you have extensive disk degeneration, bone spurs, and calcium deposits, to the point where the neck or affected section of the spine is almost fused.

The same degenerative process is also happening in the nervous system. The feedback loops we discussed in Chapter 5 are creating greater pain sensitivity, abnormal nervous system function, loss of muscle mass, and other negative effects. *The longer a subluxation is in place, the more permanent or extensive the damage to the tissues.* If left untreated, patients will progress inevitably from phase one to phase three.

Unfortunately, if patients wait too long to be treated, we run into the problem of limitations of matter. That means there is only so much recovery of function that is possible because the damage is so extensive. If a disk has become thin and lost its normal function, for instance, chiropractic won't put the disk back together again. If a nerve has been "short-circuited" for sixty years, a part of its ability to function may be lost forever. What chiropractic *can* do, however, is to produce what we call *maximum chiropractic improvement*. That means we get patients back to the highest degree of function possible, given their particular conditions and degree of subluxation damage.

The amount of time it takes to achieve maximum chiropractic improvement is almost always based on the degree of degeneration and the patient's age. As we get older, the body takes longer to heal, so a seventy-year-old will usually need more treatment than a thirty-year-old with the exact same condition. If subluxation degeneration is in phase one, we can expect a return to normal in anywhere from three to twelve months. Recovery from phase two degeneration will usually take more like twelve to twenty-four months. For someone with advanced phase three degeneration, rehabilitative care and restoring as much function as possible could take up to three years. In the Introduction I mentioned a woman named Shirley who had suffered from debilitating headaches for over fifty years. While she experienced some relief within a month or so, it took a year of treatment before the headaches were completely gone.

At the same time, it's important to note that for many patients, the relief provided by chiropractic care can be both quick and lasting. One of the great benefits of chiropractic care is that the degenerative process can be slowed down or virtually stopped because chiropractic can help stop the effects of wear and tear on the spine and nervous system. Even the smallest amount of care will make a major difference in how seniors feel, helping them regain some of their postural stability, eliminate aches and pains, and improve mental clarity and energy.

▶ Caring for Patients Who Suffer from Osteoarthritis

Our word *arthritis* comes from two Greek roots: *arthros,* "joint," and *itis,* "inflammation." Therefore *arthritis* refers to an inflammation in the joints. There are many forms of arthritis, some of which can affect the whole body, like rheumatoid or gouty arthritis. The most common form of arthritis, osteoarthritis, is a degeneration of the joints that can produce loss of cartilage, bone spurs, and pain and stiffness. Osteoarthritis frequently affects a localized area of the body, such as the neck or lower back. Joints that have been traumatized through either accident or repetitive motion injury are the most susceptible to osteoarthritis.

It is not uncommon to find that older patients who seek chiropractic care suffer from osteoarthritis of the neck and spine. Many chiropractors have found that arthritis of the spine is really the result of long-standing subluxation. As we discussed earlier, everybody has some thinning of disks and formation of bone spurs; that's part of the normal aging process. But subluxations *accelerate* the degenerative process. In fact, research points to long-standing subluxation as being a primary contributor to the development of osteoarthritis in the spine. Remember the discussion in Chapter 5 about subluxations creating an inflammatory soup in the connective tissue of the spine? It makes sense, then, that untreated subluxations could cause the very inflammation that forms the core of a diagnosis of spinal osteoarthritis. Uncorrected subluxation causes chronic inflammation in the soft tissues around the spinal joints and eventually leads to joint breakdown. This breakdown shows up as degeneration of joint spaces, thinning of disks, and formation of bone spurs.

However, regular chiropractic care can help individuals to avoid development of osteoarthritis in the spine, and if someone already has degeneration, chiropractic can slow down this process or stop it in its tracks. Chiropractic's aim is to eliminate subluxations that create inflammation in the soft tissue surrounding the spine, and reducing this inflammation often helps other joints in the body to return to normal function as well. When the body is healthy and proper nerve force is flowing throughout, patients often experience a return to a fuller range of motion, an elimination of stiffness and soreness, and more vitality in general.

When subluxations are corrected, the effects of osteoarthritis can be slowed, stopped altogether, and in some cases actually reversed. Many people with osteoarthritis experience significant relief with chiropractic, especially when it is combined with a program of gentle exercise and proper nutrition. If you suffer from osteoarthritis, or even a systemic form such as gout or rheumatoid arthritis, you can benefit from chiropractic care. However, arthritis can make the recovery process slower and more difficult than it would be for someone who has not yet developed degenerative changes. The initial relief phase of care may continue for a longer period of time, perhaps three visits per week for four to eight weeks or more. Maintenance for someone with arthritis also will be somewhat more aggressive, requiring one or two visits per month.

Many of my senior patients tell me, "Dr. Lenarz, my doctor said I shouldn't consult a chiropractor because I have osteoporosis and my bones are fragile," or "I have arthritis and the doctor says chiropractic won't help me." Whenever a senior citizen comes into my clinic, we always look for any significant osteoporosis or arthritis, as that will definitely help shape the kinds of treatment we offer. In extreme cases of osteoporosis, for instance, a very low-force chiropractic adjustment may be used; it depends on the amount of loss of bone density, where it is, and the type of adjustment needed to correct the subluxation. But patients with either osteoporosis or arthritis absolutely can receive adjustments. In some cases the condition itself will be helped by chiropractic, and in almost all cases the patient's overall health and vitality will improve.

▶ Other Benefits of Chiropractic for Seniors

Regular chiropractic care also improves patients' proprioception, or their orientation in space. This means an improvement in balance and coordination, thus eliminating one of the great fears of the elderly: falling. And since fractures, especially of the hip, can lead to a serious downward spiral in health for many senior citizens, anything that improves balance is an important part of their regular health care. I recommend my patients add some kind of gentle exercise, such as yoga or tai chi, to their routines, as both these also help strengthen muscles and improve range of motion, mobility, balance, and coordination.

Recently I went to a conference where one of the featured speakers remarked, "When people think of chiropractors, they think of a back doctor or a bone doctor. What they don't think of is a nerve doctor." But as I've said before, in truth chiropractors are primarily nervous system doctors. We treat the spine because it just happens to be the thing surrounding the nerves. So when seniors receive regular chiropractic care, one of the first things that will improve is the nervous system function. Typically people will experience improvements in digestion and elimination, as well as a general increase in the level of energy. Frequently people with emphysema, allergies, or other pulmonary-related symptoms find an improvement in their ability to breathe.

It's also fairly common for people to report improvement in conditions that they never told us about. Like Mildred and her double vision, people will come in for a treatment and say, "Oh, yeah—I noticed that since the last time I was here my eczema got better," or "My hands don't tingle anymore," or "I'm sleeping through the night for the first time in years." When we eliminate subluxations, the body can function at its best. It's even more important as we age to try to keep ourselves functioning at the highest possible level, and chiropractic care is specifically designed to help us do that.

One of the other improvements reported by patients of all ages is clearer mental functioning. Of course, there are factors that can affect mental acuity in older age that chiropractic may or may not be able to help. But I can think of three ways chiropractic care can benefit mental function. First B. J. Palmer stated that subluxations not only starve the body of proper nerve signals but also congest the brain, creating the experience of mental "fog." Eliminating subluxations seems to have an effect on both the central nervous system and certain deep recesses of the brain, helping to increase mental clarity. Second, mental functioning in the elderly often can be impeded by medications, or combinations of medications, prescribed for a range of physical ailments. As we'll discuss shortly, chiropractic's drug-free approach to health can help seniors reduce the number of medications they take, and thus eliminate a potential cause of mental confusion. Third, chiropractic at its essence is about bringing the patient back to optimal functioning. When the body functions at its best the mind will do so, too. Improving overall health is one of the best ways to keep the mind sharp as we age.

▶ Drug-Free Health Enhancement: The Promise of Chiropractic Care

In the next chapter we will talk about the incidence of iatrogenic (caused by medical treatment) disease in this country. Two of the main sources of iatrogenic disease are bad drug interactions and taking medication over a prolonged period of time. Well, a typical individual over sixty-five takes an average of three to four drugs per day, and it's not unusual to see people taking as many as five to ten prescription medications, each of them from a different specialist who doesn't really know what the patient's other doctors are prescribing. And that doesn't take into account the ever-growing list of medicines sold over the counter and taken daily by millions of people—digestive aids, laxatives, sleep aids, energy boosters, pain relievers, and so on. Is it any wonder that studies indicate that the people who suffer the most from iatrogenic disease are the elderly? Studies indicate that up to 40 percent of visits to the doctor by the elderly are for treatment of iatrogenic symptoms, often caused by bad drug interactions. To top it all off, since doctors may not be aware of all the medications the patient is taking, sometimes the doctor may prescribe yet another drug to treat the iatrogenic symptoms themselves!

The other problem with both prescription and over-the-counter medication is the length of time the patient uses them. Unfortunately, many of the conditions usually found in the elderly, such as arthritis and digestive problems, would seem to require ongoing medication. There has been a lot of publicity about the damage that taking pain relievers for too long can do to the stomach and other organs. But even the safest drugs shouldn't be consumed for too long. Taking antacids can upset the digestive balance of the stomach. Too many laxatives and the bowel loses elasticity and can't function. Too much aspirin and your stomach lining develops holes. Kidney function can be affected by long-term dosing with Tylenol. Advil and other NSAIDs can cause serious digestive problems and toxicity in the liver. When even the traditional medical establishment and the drug companies (whose business is to sell as many drugs as possible) warn against taking medication for too long, you know there's a problem. Many seniors also experience a decrease in liver function as they age. One of the liver's main roles is to remove toxins from the body, including those produced by medication. When the liver is not working well, there can be a dangerous buildup of chemicals in the body—yet another reason for seniors to avoid medications when at all possible.

Chiropractic and alternative health care are vital for the elderly as well as the population at large. Any treatment that can decrease our dependence on drugs, offer us increased vitality and improved functioning, and restore our zest for living is an invaluable support for our health. Certainly some medications may be needed, depending on the condition of the patient and the extent of damage to the body. But if you look one by one at the typical complaints of our senior citizens, I'll bet that 80 to 90 percent of them can be helped, if not cured, by alternative means. What's more important, since alternative care such as chiropractic is about increasing health, not healing disease, the "side effects" of such care are usually only positive. Instead of less mental clarity, people experience more. Instead of lowered vitality and energy, people feel better, look better, and can do more. Instead of having to worry about the effects of combining medications, people can rest assured they are working with their bodies to create the greatest degree of health possible.

A few years ago I had a lovely elderly patient whom I'd been seeing about once a month. She'd just turned ninety and things weren't working quite as well as they used to. She was starting to stoop over, she was having trouble walking, and in general she wasn't feeling good. She told me, "Goodness, I'm only ninety and I feel like I'm ninety-five!" Now, a lot of people would just chalk her symptoms up to extreme old age, but I talked to her and asked her to try coming in once a week for a while. After a few months she was able to walk into my office unassisted. She was standing much straighter, and said she was feeling much better—"I feel like I'm eighty-five again!" she told me. Now, feeling eighty-five might not sound that good to you, but for this lady it was wonderful. She had gotten her mobility back, and she had more energy. Instead of using the excuse of old age, this lady was doing all she could to feel her best for as long as possible. And isn't that what we all want as we reach the end of life?

PART III

A New Model
of Health Care

14

Why We Need a New Model of Health Care

Jeannie, a patient of mine in her mid-thirties, came to me one day and explained that she was suffering from vertigo. Vertigo is a sensation of faintness or dizziness where a person feels as though his or her surroundings are spinning. Jeannie's attacks occurred mostly at night when she was in bed, but they were unpredictable and could occur at any time during the day as well. The experience left her feeling nauseated, fatigued, and anxious—and fearful of a dangerous fall or auto accident.

Jeannie related that she had gone to a medical doctor and been told that her problem most likely resulted from a "loose hair" in her inner ear. The doctor didn't offer any solution except the hope that the hair might settle into a stationary position on its own, relieving her of her symptoms. After an examination I found that her upper neck was out of adjustment. With just one adjustment the vertigo diminished by about 75 percent. After the second adjustment, two days later, the problem resolved completely. The dramatic improvement that resulted from correcting her subluxation led me to question the validity of the medical diagnosis.

But then a new problem began to emerge. Because her vertigo had been very intense and happened mostly in bed at night, Jeannie began to develop an anxiety problem. Even though the vertigo was gone, her fear of its return led to a feeling of nervousness every night when trying to sleep. She started to develop chronic nighttime anxiety, which was accompanied by occasional night sweats, nausea, and abdominal cramping. She went back to her M.D., who diagnosed depression and prescribed an antidepressant (a typical scenario). The antidepressant seemed to work for a couple of weeks, but then Jeannie's body adapted to the drug and her symptoms returned. She went back to her medical doctor once again and he prescribed a stronger antidepressant. She was to start off with one pill before going to bed and over the next few days build up to two pills per day. She was warned of some possible side effects but was not prepared for what the first night would hold.

Jeannie took the prescription on Friday evening. She described it as a night from hell. She was up the entire night, experiencing intense anxiety, restlessness, and severe hallucinations. Her husband told her the next morning that at one point during the long night she said, "There are spiderwebs coming out of my mouth." Over the weekend she suffered with confusion and anxiety, and even had difficulty speaking. It took two days for her to begin to feel somewhat normal again. She didn't take any more of the pills, and spoke with her M.D. on Monday. After she explained her reaction to the prescription, the doctor asked if she had followed his instructions to increase the dose to two pills!

Unfortunately, the story continues. As Jeannie was telling me this, I said to her, "It sounds as if there might be some hormonal problems here." She replied that this was her mother's opinion as well. Jeannie decided to return to her M.D. and express this concern. He agreed that might be the case and ran a series of tests to investigate further. He counseled her that if this was a hormonal imbalance, there were two surgical options to correct the problem: arthroscopic surgery to singe the inside wall of the uterus (thus leaving it nonfunctional) or complete removal of her ovaries.

Jeannie came back to me, understandably upset. From vertigo to a recommendation of having her ovaries removed in less than two months! I was, quite frankly, appalled at the whole series of events and recommendations. Given her current symptoms, my first suggestion was to explore areas of the spine that had nerves going to the hormone-producing organs and possibly other abdominal areas. I took new X rays of the spine and did a full spinal examination. I discovered some problem areas and adjusted the locations that showed nerve interference due to subluxation. I also recommended that she seek the help of a massage therapist who specialized in abdominal work, and to consult a naturopath. As it turned out, the adjustments fully resolved all the symptoms within two weeks.

Jeannie's story exemplifies the often confusing and difficult experience of being a health care consumer. According to a survey conducted by the Harvard School of Public Health in 1994, only 18 percent of those questioned were satisfied with the American health care system. Unfortunately, Jeannie's experience is similar to that of hundreds of thousands of Americans per year who become ill as a result of following the directions of their medical doctor. More often than not, this problem arises from harmful drug reactions and interactions. But the problem doesn't stop there. It turns into a more serious and dark affair when you look at the worst-case scenarios that result from the problems of our current health care system.

I was first alerted to one of our most alarming health care problems long before I became a chiropractor. It was 1976, and I was reading the *Pittsburgh Post-Gazette*. The article was buried deep in the newspaper, on one of those pages that is 90 percent advertisement and 10 percent news. A one-paragraph article, perhaps six sentences long, announced that a study had found that almost a hundred thousand people a year were dying from a serious health problem, iatrogenic disease. What *was* this, and why wasn't it front-page news? In the intervening years, I have studied many research articles on different aspects of iatrogenic disease. I also became a chiropractor, and I now examine this information from the perspective of chiropractic's philosophy of restoring health rather than treating symptoms.

Iatro is a Greek root that means "physician," and *genic* means "created." Therefore, iatrogenic disease is physician-created illness—health problems that are caused by medical care and which can even result in death. *Iatrogenic disease is one of the top five causes of death in the United States.* Here are a few statistics collected by some of conventional medicine's top organizations.

- In *To Err Is Human: Building a Safer Health System,* a 1999 report authored by the Committee on Quality of Health Care in America and published by the Institute of Medicine (a non-profit organization under the auspices of the National Academy of Sciences, mandated by the U.S. Congress to provide health policy advice to the government), reviewers said hospital errors kill anywhere from 44,000 to 98,000 patients a year. "Even using the lower estimate," the report states, "preventable medical errors in hospitals exceed deaths attributable to such feared threats as motor-vehicle wrecks, breast cancer, and AIDS." Errors included adverse drug reactions, transfusion errors, surgical injuries (including wrong-site surgeries), restraint-related injuries, falls, burns, pressure sores, and mistaken patient identities.

- A 1995–96 study published in the *Journal of the American Medical Association* reviewed patient deaths at seven Veterans Administration medical centers. It concluded, "Similar to previous studies, almost a quarter (22.7 percent) of active-care patient deaths were rated as at least possibly preventable by optimal care, with 6.0 percent rated as probably or definitely preventable." However, the study went on to state that this figure would be much lower if patients were evaluated based on whether they would have lived three months or more after they left the hospital, and whether they would have had "good physical and cognitive functioning." (I don't know about you, but if my father had died from less than optimal hospital care, the doctor telling me, "Well, he wouldn't have lived that much longer anyway" wouldn't be much consolation.)

- A seminal 1984 study conducted by a team of Harvard physicians (the Harvard Medical Practice Study) and published in the *New England Journal of Medicine* evaluated thirty thousand hospitalization records from New York State. They found that 18 percent of drug complications were due to negligence. In addition, 75 percent of cases of improper or delayed diagnosis were due to negligence. Adverse events due to negligence occurred more frequently in the elderly. The authors extrapolated that "among the 2.7 million hospitalizations in New York in 1984, adverse events occurred in nearly 99,000 hospitalizations, and 14 percent of these led to death."

- In 2000 the *Archives of Internal Medicine* published an article that reviewed current medical literature on increased risk for older patients (over sixty-five years old) for injuries associated with hospitalization. Possible injuries were divided into six categories: adverse drug reactions, falls, infections acquired at the hospital, pressure sores, delirium, and complications before, during, and after surgery. They concluded that "for each of these categories, older patients appear to be at greater risk, ranging from a 2.2-fold increase for [surgical] complications to a 10-fold increase for falling." They added, "Many of these complications appear to be preventable."

- Speaking of surgery, in 2002 the *Archives of Surgery* reported a study at a university teaching hospital of procedures done at four different surgical services: general surgery, combined general surgery and trauma, vascular surgery, and cardiothoracic surgery. Their findings: "Despite mortality rates that compare favorably with national benchmarks, a prospective examination of surgical patients reveals complication rates that are 2 to 4 times higher than those identified in an Institute of Medicine report. Almost half of these adverse events were judged contemporaneously by peers to be due to provider error (avoidable). Errors in care contributed to 38 (30%) of 128 deaths."

- Finally, according to a study published in 2002 in the *Annual Review of Public Health,* during the years 1983 to 1998 U.S. fatalities from acknowledged prescription errors increased by 243 percent. "This percentage increase was greater than for almost any other cause of death, and far outpaced the increase in the number of prescriptions." Of course, it doesn't help that the number of prescriptions has risen from 1.5 billion in 1989 to a projected 3 billion in 2000, according to the National Association of Chain Drug Stores.

Although medicine has done many wonders for humankind, it also has a dark side. There are serious problems with the very foundation upon which medicine is based. The epidemic problem of iatrogenic deaths is one of the symptoms of this problem. This is one of the reasons that I decided to become a chiropractor. I saw that there were grave problems in medicine, and that chiropractic was the largest drug-free healing profession in the world. I also saw that much of our culture was living in denial of the basic flaws of traditional medicine. How could a hundred thousand people a year be dying from *any* cause without there being vigorous public debate about the problem?

▶ History of Modern Medicine: How Did We Get Here?

Germ theory—the idea that germs exist and cause illness—was first written about in the sixteenth and seventeenth centuries. The first use of vaccination was discovered and promoted by Edward Jenner in England in the late 1700s. By the mid-1800s, Louis Pasteur's work brought the germ theory to maturity by demonstrating its relevance "to infectious disease, surgery, hospital management, agriculture and industry." Another key player during that time, Robert Koch, created the basis for the scientific investigation of germs and the diseases they cause. Many of his techniques are still used today.

Other medical advances in the nineteenth century were the discovery of anesthesia and proper surgical hygiene. Hygiene was of course tied to an understanding of germs. It was Joseph Lister who developed the "antiseptic system" to reduce hospital infections. This system involved washing of hands between patients (especially when the physician was dealing with open wounds) and the use of antiseptics and sterilization techniques. Anesthesia allowed surgery to be performed without excruciating pain for the first time in history. Penicillin, discovered by Alexander Fleming in 1928, was the "magic bullet" that could kill the germ without harming the individual.

These advances built the foundation of what we call modern medicine, with its reliance on drug therapy. Medical societies and the pharmaceutical industry grew in power and prestige, developing yet more powerful tools. It seemed as though there was nothing that medicine could not achieve.

And yet, with all of these wonderful achievements, how did

medicine end up in the crisis we see today? How do we explain or understand the problems of soaring medical costs and epidemic illness caused by medical care? The enigmatic problem of iatrogenic disease makes it impossible to point a finger at one particular cause. If there *is* something understandable about iatrogenesis, it is that there are a wide variety of causes. Medicine defends itself by declaring that since it works with sick people who have an impossibly wide scope of diseases, and because the art of medicine is always developing, inevitably there are going to be people who either die or get sicker while medicine attempts to help them.

Although this argument certainly has its validity, there are some disturbing facts that compel us to investigate further. In his book *Confessions of a Medical Heretic,* Robert Mendelsohn, M.D., reveals some distressing incidents. For instance, in 1974 in Israel, medical doctors went on strike. But according to the Jerusalem Burial Society, during the strike the death rate in Israel dropped 50 percent! As soon as the strike was over, however, the death rate went back to its previous level. Drops in death rates also were seen during a physicians strike in Bogotá, Colombia, in 1974, and with a work slowdown in Los Angeles County in 1976. How can this be? Are doctors saving lives or taking them?

Thomas McKeown, emeritus professor of social medicine at the University of Birmingham in England, wrote a book called *The Role of Medicine: Dream, Mirage, or Nemesis.* Although the book does not delve at any length into iatrogenesis, McKeown does present an in-depth examination of the role medicine has played in reducing death and illness in our society. He asks the question, "Are we living longer, and are we less sick, as a result of modern medicine?" His answer to both these questions is no. He proves through historical and statistical analysis that the increase in how long we live and the decrease in the rate of disease are almost wholly due to changes in *environmental* factors rather than medical treatment. Clean water, proper food-handling practices, proper hygiene, and lifestyle changes are the main causes of increased health and longer life in Western society.

So, what has medicine done for humanity? McKeown indicates that medicine has indeed accounted for a few percentage points of improved health and longevity. And of course we all know someone who has been helped by medicine. Perhaps your own life may have been saved by medical intervention. Although it may seem that I am critical of medicine, I wouldn't want to live in a world where medicine didn't exist. I believe the issue is not to eliminate good medicine but to find out what is good in medicine and what is bad, what needs to stay and what needs to go.

As I have studied chiropractic, healing, public health, and iatrogenic disease, it has become exceedingly clear to me that there is a need for new leadership in health care. Chiropractic philosophy sets the foundation for a safer, saner model of health care that will take us into the new century. Already the tide is turning, and because chiropractors have been quietly healing people for over a hundred years—teaching these foundational principles while bringing health to millions upon millions—chiropractors stand at the crossroads, ready to usher in a new age of health care.

Unfortunately, chiropractors and medical doctors all too often have been at odds. This serves neither conventional medicine nor chiropractic. Nor, ultimately, does it benefit the patient, who seeks only to get better and usually doesn't care how the cure occurs. Patients are best served by *cooperation* between health care providers, not by animosity and lack of communication. Indeed, the counterbalance of differing opinions and methods is valuable because it gives people greater choice. When conventional and alternative medical practitioners work together, the patient's needs can be addressed at a much higher level, producing better health and increased satisfaction with the level of care offered. I have seen such treatment in action. In fact, I am currently working with a group of physicians to develop a cooperative D.C./M.D. practice where a number of conventional and alternative practitioners will work together.

The key, I believe, is to allow conventional medicine to do what it does best: handle serious trauma and treat life-threatening disease. Conventional medicine has made great strides in overcoming infectious disease and treating many types of cancer as well as genetic problems such as sickle cell anemia and hemophilia. It also shines in its ability to provide early diagnosis and treatment of diseases before they become more serious and life-threatening. Today there are hundreds of relatively simple screening processes for many diseases, and early detection can increase the chances of successful treatment. Indeed, the growing focus on early detection has moved conventional medicine toward a more preventive approach to health care. And from a focus on prevention, it is only a short step to the newest movement in conventional medical care: health promotion. Leaders of the health promotion movement—M.D.'s such as Deepak Chopra, Bernie Siegel, and Andrew Weil—have begun to adopt a chiropractic-like philosophy based on the concept of the inner wisdom of the body. There is a growing awareness of the body's ability to heal itself and of the need to avoid dangerous diagnostic and treatment procedures if safer, saner approaches are available. Many patients are in agreement with this approach, and they are looking for conventional medical practitioners who are open to recommending whatever medical option will produce the best results in terms of both cure rate and quality of life. In today's health care climate, there is no doubt that cooperation between practitioners serves the patient's needs best.

▶ Health Care or Disease Care?

I ask all of my patients to attend a class when they begin care. At that class I pose two questions about our current health care system. The first is: "How much money does your medical doctor make on a healthy patient?" The second is similar: "How much money do the pharmaceutical companies make on a healthy patient?" The answer to both questions is the same: little to none. We don't have a system that profits from health; we have a system that profits from disease. Allopathic medicine tends to treat the body's illnesses rather than promote its health. Because conventional medicine focuses primarily on treating illness, it can be called more accurately a disease care system rather than a health care system. I cannot utilize the conventional medical system until I am in a state of breakdown—until there are signs and symptoms for my doctor to treat. Medical doctors rarely, if ever, look at a healthy patient and ask, "How can medicine increase this person's health and vitality?"

Certainly conventional medicine is making some effort toward what it calls "promoting health," but mostly what that really means is catching disease earlier. Medicine's current and growing focus on well-baby checkups, blood pressure and cholesterol screening, mammograms, colon cancer screenings, prostate exams, and bone density tests, for example, is valuable. But while early detection is a move in the right direction, it is still based on the disease care model.

Now, don't get me wrong: As I've said, I'm glad that we have a disease care system. Conventional medicine is unmatched in its ability to diagnose and treat severe illness and trauma. This system helps countless millions, but it has also become blind to its own deficiencies. In its desire to intervene and its certainty that it will provide the best treatment available in every circumstance, it has betrayed its own fundamental principle of "First, do no harm." This is evident in the fact that somewhere around a hundred thousand people every year are killed by the system that is meant to save their lives.

What is the root cause of this problem? What can be done so that we can become better health care consumers and avoid some of the dangers of medicine? What can be done to help the whole system move forward? To answer these questions, we need to look at some of the fundamental principles upon which modern medicine is based.

First, what is it that medical doctors do? I believe the following is a broad and fair definition: *Medical doctors diagnose and treat symptoms, disease, and trauma.* But there are limitations to this type of care. To use an analogy most people can relate to, let's say I bought a new car. (I usually buy used cars, but this time I've bought a brand-new Ford Mustang.) I want this car to last a long time—at least ten years. Now, I need to make it clear that I drive a *lot*. Over the last five years I have driven a minimum of thirty-five thousand miles per year. (This comes with opening and managing a number of chiropractic offices in the region.) For the sake of the example, let's also say that I decide to put some restrictions on how my new car will be cared for. No one is allowed to change the oil. No one is allowed to tune up the car. Not even me. No one is even allowed to open the hood. Do you think my new car will last ten years? Of course not. Without any maintenance, and with the number of miles that I drive on a yearly basis, I'll be lucky if it lasts a few years.

Let's take this example a little further. Suppose I have been driving my new car for three years and it runs out of oil. I am driving down the highway and my engine freezes up. I have my car towed to the mechanic and I tell him, "Please hurry up and fix this. I have an important meeting in fifteen minutes." The mechanic will take a quick look at my engine and say, "You're not getting this car back in fifteen minutes. I have to replace the whole engine."

Driving a car into the ground with no maintenance sounds pretty silly, doesn't it? But isn't that often how we treat our health? We drive ourselves until we break down, then we run to the doctor and say, "Fix me now, please. I'm in a hurry. I don't have time to heal because I have places to go and people to see." We wait until we are in a state of physical or mental breakdown before we do anything about our health. We wait until we are in crisis before we take our health seriously. This is called crisis care. And unfortunately, it's what we have come to regard as the normal approach to health care in this country.

This attitude is our real health care crisis. The system of disease care is all about crisis: intervention once we have broken down. Any system that habitually operates in crisis mode will have two primary characteristics. First, the system will be very expensive.

After all, crisis usually means significant damage has already been done, and therefore the patients will cost more to treat. Second, and far worse, it is more than likely that mistakes will be made. Crisis often requires quick and massive intervention—broad-spectrum antibiotics, surgical solutions, and other invasive procedures. In its haste to heal, medicine can find itself curing the disease but killing the patient.

Chiropractic, on the other hand, stands firmly in the school of thought that promotes the expression of health rather than treatment of disease. While many people initially seek out chiropractic for treatment of symptoms, chiropractic is really about facilitating the full expression of Innate Intelligence, the full expression of life. As we enter the twenty-first century, people of the world are beginning to understand what chiropractors have been saying for a hundred years: that although there is a need for disease care, there is even a greater need for health care. We don't need care that just treats and prevents disease, but also care that promotes health and the full expression of life. Although chiropractic care can help those in certain types of crisis, it is better used as a means of maintenance of health throughout life.

▶ The AMA and Chiropractic

In 1976 Chester Wilk, D.C., and four other chiropractors filed a restraint-of-trade suit against the American Medical Association (AMA). At the time, the AMA referred to chiropractors as "quacks" and refused to recognize them as legitimate health care providers. The suit, *Wilk et al. vs. AMA,* wound its long, tortuous way through the courts until September 1987, when a federal district court in Chicago found the AMA and others guilty of illegal conspiracy, restraint of trade, and antitrust violations in relation to its activities against the chiropractic profession. The court ordered a permanent injunction against the AMA, forcing them to print the court's findings in the *Journal of the American Medical Association.*

Several other defendants settled out of court, helping to pay for the chiropractors' legal expenses and making donations to Kentuckiana Children's Center, a chiropractic nonprofit home for disabled children. The court's decision was upheld in the U.S. Court of Appeals under Judge Susan Getzendanner in 1990, and again by the U.S. Supreme Court that same year.

Even with the success of the Wilk case and other antitrust litigation, the AMA continues to this day to wage a campaign against chiropractic. Today the attacks take the form of overstated concerns about the safety of chiropractic health care. The truth is that chiropractic has proven itself over the last hundred-plus years to be safe and effective.

I have never been a proponent of conspiracy theories, but I recently had a patient ask me rhetorically, "Dr. Lenarz, if you had all the power and all the money, wouldn't you want to keep it?" Is this why the medical industry has fought chiropractic so bitterly for so long?

What we view as medicine today is a system that developed over twenty-five hundred years but has recently taken a turn that is both miraculous and terrifying. Medicine is miraculous in its ability to cure infectious disease, treat trauma, and save the lives of those on the brink of death. But the flip side of the miracle is the epidemic incidence of iatrogenic disease and death. The medical industry is a multinational conglomeration of powerful corporations (primarily pharmaceutical companies), trade and professional organizations, government and educational institutions, and special-interest groups. It is a ship of gigantic proportions. Unfortunately, in many ways it is a ship out of control. The decision by Judge Getzendanner specifically stated that the AMA was motivated by economic self-interest in its attempt to shut down chiropractic, not by an interest in the health of the public. I am a strong believer in the marketplace, but when economic self-interest begins to affect the health of people around the world, something must change.

Chiropractic has stepped into this fray as a drug-free alternative that threatens the very basis of medicine. In large part medicine has led us to believe that health comes from a bottle and that the answers to mankind's oldest problems—death and disease—are only a step away. Just $1 billion more for the development of this pill, they tell us; just another billion for the development of this genetically altered substance, just a few more billions in research funded by public money and the pharmaceutical industry, and we will have no more disease. But as one new cure arises, so do a dozen new diseases. Just like Gilgamesh (whom you met in Chapter 3), it seems we stand at the threshold of great discovery only to realize that the life-giving herb has slipped from our grasp.

The things that truly advance humanity are rare. Certainly medicine has made great contributions, but as the research of McKeown and others has shown, the most widespread health advancements for all of us have come from simple changes in public health policy. Things such as clean water, proper disposal of waste, and better nutrition have strengthened our health as a society. But I believe that chiropractic practice, coupled with chiropractic philosophy, can provide another great advancement in the health and well-being of humankind. Indeed, the precepts that chiropractic has been based on, and which chiropractors have been teaching for over a hundred years, are starting to weave themselves deeply into the fabric of everyday life in America and many other countries throughout the world.

▶ The Foundation of Health

Chiropractors who promote an understanding of Innate Intelligence and the power of adjustment have often been accused of saying that chiropractic is a cure-all. But the idea that chiropractors are saying they can heal everything is a misconception. While a healthy spine and nervous system are foundational to good health, they are not a panacea. So how is it that chiropractic and chiropractic philosophy fit into the broader picture of health and disease care? How is it that the correction of subluxation and the teaching of chiropractic philosophy place chiropractors in the leadership position they enjoy today with such a large percentage of the population? There are basically two reasons for this. Correction of subluxation is foundational to creating health, and chiropractic philosophy is foundational to understanding health. While medicine has focused for twenty-five hundred years on the treatment of disease, chiropractic is focused on the causes of health.

Here's what I mean by foundational. At best a person can live for about forty to sixty days without food, four to ten days without water, only a few minutes without air. We would all agree that food, water, and air are foundational to life, correct? These are all external things we are dependent upon for our existence. In a similar way, chiropractic deals with the *internal* functioning that is foundational to life. Most of us never stop to think about it, but how long could we live without our brain being attached to our body? Not even a few minutes! We don't have to run expensive research projects to know that the brain needs to be attached to the body for the body to function properly. Just like food, air, and water, the mental impulses that travel from the brain down the spinal cord and out over the nerves are also foundational to life.

When the brain gets disconnected from the body, life stops immediately. This is because the brain and spinal cord control and coordinate all body functions. And, as discussed in detail in Chapter 3, the brain is the incarnation of Innate Intelligence. Even though every cell in the body has infinite wisdom within it, the organism (the human being) as a whole has a seat of intelligence: the brain. If the brain is disconnected, the body becomes very stupid very fast! When we get a subluxation, it's a little bit like being disconnected. Subluxation begins to cut off the brain's ability to fully communicate with the body. Subluxations interfere with the very foundation of proper physiological functioning. Therefore, chiropractic adjustments, which restore proper communication between the brain and the body, are foundational to health.

We may have a great exercise routine, a positive mental attitude, and a healthy diet. But if our brain is even slightly disconnected from our body, we can never express health fully. We can never digest food fully if nerves going to our stomach and intestines are short-circuited. No matter how much we exercise, if the nerves going to our heart and lungs are subluxated, our cardiovascular health can be diminished. This is not to say that exercise and a good diet are not important, but rather to illustrate that *normal physiological function is dependent on a properly functioning nervous system.* This is why chiropractic adjustments are foundational to health.

There are other things that are foundational to our health as well. There are choices we make that can help our body to perform at a higher level. For instance, cardiovascular exercise can improve the health of our lungs, heart, and circulation, which in turn can affect many aspects of our health. As noted in Chapter 9, nutrition can also affect our health dramatically. For every system in our body, from the nervous system to the immune system and the circulatory system, there are things we can do to enhance their performance.

If we look at the body from the perspective of systems, then we can work to ensure that every system is performing at its best. When we look at creating health in this way, we are acknowledging that we are not victims but instead have a say in our health and well-being. We also are placing ourselves squarely on one side of a debate between differing schools of thought in healing that has been going on for centuries. One school of thought says that the doctor's primary job is to treat *disease.* The other school believes that the primary job of the doctor is to treat the *patient.* Although both of these approaches have merit, let's take a look at what this debate is all about.

When we talk about treating a disease, the disease usually is viewed as an entity unto itself, one that needs to be fought and conquered, like overcoming an infection or cancer. Doctors who treat disease will do everything they can to fight it, even if the treatment is equally (if not more) dangerous than the illness being treated. The disease fighter looks at health as coming from the outside in, and usually will fight illness with drugs and surgery. A doctor using the other approach, which focuses on treating the patient, would say, "We need to strengthen the patient, build up her immune system and overall ability to fight illness. Then the body's own defenses will heal her." The patient-focused doctor looks at health as coming from the inside out, and has historically taken care of patients with diet, exercise, and adjustments.

▶ Chiropractic and Medicine: Inside Out and Outside In

For most of the twentieth century, conventional medical doctors would have nothing to do with chiropractors, whom they viewed as quacks. Conversely, most chiropractors considered medical doctors to be butchers and drug dealers. But as with most things in this world, the truth lies somewhere in the middle. Chiropractic has survived because it has helped enough people to have powerful grassroots support. Medicine has survived because of its success in helping people as well. Perhaps both professions have survived in part because they are filled with individuals of strong will and determination.

Regardless of the reasons, medicine and chiropractic have had to learn to coexist. In many cases this relationship has flourished; in other circumstances the relationship is strained at best. But I believe it is important for you, the health care consumer, to know how to use both chiropractic and medicine wisely in your life. It is also important for you to understand the value of applying chiropractic principles in the wider health care arena. If properly understood and applied, chiropractic philosophy can help you to make better health care decisions. When applied on a societal level, chiropractic philosophy can change the face of health care worldwide.

What are the strengths of the medical approach? What are the strengths of the chiropractic approach? How can these two differing viewpoints come together to make a better world for all of us?

If I was in a serious auto accident and ended up on the side of the road with grave internal injuries and severe bleeding, the last person I would want to see at that point would be my chiropractor! There can be little debate about the strength of medicine in treating traumatic injury. Medicine does this, and many other things, very well. But there are a lot of things that medicine does *not* do well, such as prevention, and often treatment, of chronic diseases. And as noted earlier, sometimes the treatment conventional medicine offers is more harmful than the disease. As consumers and as a society, we have to be willing to take a hard look at what works and doesn't work in medicine. Is our condition best treated by the crisis response of conventional medicine? Or are there other options we should explore that will provide more appropriate care?

As individuals, you and I also need to look hard at the practitioners we choose to work with. Medicine is an art, not a science— an art that uses the tools of science, but an art nonetheless. While we tend to think of medicine as a science that is applied consistently, in reality we can go to five different doctors with the same problem and come up with five different diagnoses! Even if we came up with just one diagnosis, we could be given five different treatment plans. This is why we need to take responsibility for our own health and become aware health care consumers.

Chiropractic philosophy would ask three questions of anyone seeking help with an illness.

1. *Have you ruled out the possibility that subluxation is at the root of the problem?* Correction of subluxation is noninvasive and a powerful healing modality.

2. *Have you discovered what is interfering with the expression of Innate Intelligence and hence with your basic physiological functioning?* Is it subluxation? Is it a nutritional imbalance? Is it some toxicity? Is it chronic sadness or depression?

3. *What is the least invasive way to solve your health problem?* Chiropractic philosophy would always support the procedure or choice that would solve the problem with the least amount of danger to you. This is the simple logic of chiropractic philosophy.

If these three basic questions were asked about all your health problems, and the time were taken to work through these steps with both chiropractors and medical doctors, the quality of health care in your life would improve dramatically. If these simple three questions were asked on a national or global basis, it could create a saner and safer health care model the world over.

It may seem a little silly to ask whether correcting a subluxation would make any difference to someone with cancer or could possibly affect a problem as serious as the AIDS epidemic in Africa. But in reality, correction of subluxation has been shown to increase the strength of the immune system in both the short term and the long run. Although not necessarily effecting a cure, a strengthened immune system certainly could influence outcomes in both AIDS and cancer patients. In many cases, however, chiropractic can stand on its own in both the cure and prevention of many health problems. It can also be a potent ally when used in conjunction with either alternative or traditional medical treatments.

Once again this brings us around to one of the greatest strengths of chiropractic: *When used as a means of maintenance of health, chiropractic correction of subluxation can increase both the quality and the length of life.* Chiropractic is not only a means of health care or even a philosophy; it can also be a lifestyle. The chiropractic lifestyle is based on living subluxation-free and allowing Innate Intelligence to express itself fully. It understands that drugs are toxic and dangerous and should be used sparingly; it teaches children that they are complete within themselves and don't need drugs to feel good. It is a lifestyle that embraces the choices that increase your chances for health. Ultimately, it is a lifestyle that welcomes the complete and full expression of life.

15

Walking Your Own Path to Radiant Health: Choosing the Method of Healing That's Right for You

Although I do believe there are fundamental flaws in the current medical system, I am more interested in you, the patient, getting the best care possible and becoming a well-educated health care consumer. This goes far beyond choosing the right HMO or the best doctor; it has to do with your fundamental health philosophy. Your principles will guide your choices on everything from diet to exercise to doctors to supplements to drugs to ongoing care.

If you choose to ignore your health until you become ill and see a medical practitioner only when you get to the point of breakdown, then perhaps the world of conventional medicine alone will suit you. But I believe most of us would rather be healthy and alive instead of just "not sick." The statistics on the number of people who take supplements, exercise, go on diets designed to promote weight loss and greater health, and seek alternative medical treatments (at last count, over 50 percent of the population) demonstrate to me that people want to be healthy.

Chiropractic clearly can be part of a health maintenance program and is not limited to general health improvement. As you've seen so far, chiropractic has helped millions of people with a wide variety of health problems. Keep in mind the major premise of chiropractic: *Health is our natural state.*

Even though you are surrounded by the power of the conventional medical system (with its multibillion-dollar companies, its tie-ins with the government, and its seeming fear of allowing patients to try other options that the system cannot control or profit from), ultimately you are the one responsible for your own health. Choose the philosophy of health that makes the most sense to you, then choose health care that will be in tune with your true understanding.

Your next decision is to create a plan for supporting your health. Within the conventional medical system, patients usually have a primary physician and, depending on their disease and/or condition, a specialist or team of specialists who are experts in treating specific areas of the body. Patients also have a wide range of health insurance plans to choose from, depending on how much they can afford to spend and what services they wish to access. Within the alternative medicine system, you also can choose a team of specialists to support your ongoing health and vitality. This would include your chiropractor, dentist, naturopath, and nutritionist, and perhaps your massage therapist or exercise teacher. Some people might consider such services a luxury rather than a necessity. But again, it depends on your attitude toward health. As we discussed in the previous chapter, an investment in alternative health care is an investment in health maintenance and disease prevention.

So let's say that as a health care consumer, you have decided to have it both ways: to use alternative medicine as a means of ongoing health promotion, and to have conventional medicine as your fallback in case of trauma or severe illness. And let's say you experience some sort of physical dis-ease (literally, a lack of ease—everything from lowered vitality to specific symptoms). Your first question should be, "What am I seeking help for?" In the case of acute pain, trauma, or severe illness, the needs are very immediate. Although chiropractic can help with some crises, such as back and neck pain, crisis is one of the areas of strength for conventional medicine. When it comes to chronic problems, however, or general feelings of lack of energy or malaise, usually I suggest that the patient see me first. Quite frankly, one of the reasons I make this recommendation is that chiropractors rarely hesitate to refer patients to conventional medical doctors, while it's not true the other way around. No matter what, the care offered by chiropractic will do no harm and will probably increase the patient's overall health—and that can only be to the good.

▶ Choosing Your Health Care Practitioner

Here are some suggestions for evaluating and selecting your health care practitioners, whether they specialize in conventional or alternative medicine.

1. **Find a doctor who is both a teacher and a clinician.** The word *doctor* is derived from the Latin *docere,* to teach. In the world of higher education, a doctor is someone who has received a doctorate and is now a teacher or professor. The degree that a medical doctor receives is a doctorate of medicine; the degree that a chiropractor receives is a doctorate of chiropractic.

   When I choose a health care professional, I want a doctor who is both an excellent teacher and an excellent clinician. I consider the roles to be equally important. Why? Because the role of making health care choices ultimately lies with the patient, not the doctor, and it is only through teaching that doctors empower patients to take responsibility for their own health. It is the doctor's responsibility to give the patient all the information required to make a wise decision. In the end, the patient may refer that responsibility back to the doctor, but even this decision ought to be based on complete and understandable information.

2. **Insist on good communication**. Good communication between patient and doctor has the same qualities that we see in any healthy team, whether it be husband and wife, parent and child, or a pair of friends. These qualities include give-and-take, honesty, and clarity. Interestingly, I have seen that the quality of the doctor-patient relationship is not necessarily a matter of spending a lot of time together on each visit. It starts with the desire for a great relationship on both sides. The doctor must bring to the relationship an ability not only to be thorough in his or her clinical and scientific assessment, but also to clearly communicate necessary information to the patient. But it is the patient's responsibility to be equally clear and concise in his or her communication, and to demand excellence of the doctor. If there is ever a doubt or concern that you leave unexpressed, the doctor cannot read your mind. You need to ask your questions clearly and request answers that you can fully understand.

3. **Insist on playing an active part in your health care decisions.** When either the patient or the doctor relinquishes responsibility for these very basic "team rules," the quality of the relationship—and therefore the quality of the care—is reduced. Jeannie's story in the previous chapter is an example of a serious breakdown in the doctor-patient relationship. Perhaps her doctor's clinical assessment, diagnosis, and treatment were off base. But doctors are human, which means they can learn. Going back to her medical doctor, explaining what had happened, and engaging him in a conversation about the possibility of hormonal imbal-

ances made Jeannie a more active participant in her own health care. It challenged the doctor to listen to the patient and question his own perception, which led to a different diagnosis and care recommendation. Jeannie then took that information and sought out alternative forms of therapy that helped her to resolve her problems. Jeannie took on the task of actively gathering information. She also took it upon herself to ask different practitioners about their opinions regarding her condition. This is active and smart consumer behavior.

4. **Even if you receive a diagnosis from a conventional medical doctor, feel free to try alternative medicine to treat your condition.** One of the strengths of medicine is not only its treatment of trauma but also its diagnostic capabilities. But this is a double-edged sword for the consumer. Just because conventional medical doctors can tell you what's going on, do you necessarily want them to treat your condition? Remember, your choices in conventional medicine are limited to two fundamentals: drugs or surgery (with an occasional lifestyle recommendation thrown in). In many cases, however, the treatment recommended carries with it unwanted consequences. Or perhaps it's just not in alignment with your basic philosophy of health. As a consumer, you can decide whether you wish to take the treatment recommendation or seek other means of care.

I had an acquaintance who came back from a trip abroad with very bad chest congestion. She was somewhat worried, because she was returning from an extended stay in a third-world country. As a child she had had bronchitis several times, and her family had a history of sensitivity in the lungs. But she also believed strongly in the body's ability to heal itself. So she went to see her family's conventional medical doctor. He listened to her chest and said, "You have an upper respiratory infection. I'm going to prescribe an antibiotic for you."

"Do I have bronchitis or pneumonia?" she asked the doctor.

"No," he told her. "Just an upper respiratory infection."

"Thank you," she said, and left. The diagnosis had given her peace of mind, and she was certain her body could heal an upper respiratory infection by itself. She never filled the prescription; instead, she went to bed and kept herself well hydrated and warm. In three days she was back to normal. My acquaintance had used conventional medicine's diagnostic abilities to give her some peace of mind about her illness. Then she made the choice to rely on means other than taking a drug to heal herself. She also could have used alternative medicine to support her in restoring her health through natural means.

5. **If your alternative care isn't providing you with the results you want over a period of time, feel free to seek other methods of treating your condition.** The responsibility of the patient to decide on the most appropriate treatment holds equally true when the patient prefers to use alternative medicine as the first option. Let's say someone comes to see me complaining of headaches. I begin by checking the spine for nerve interference. I find subluxations, I adjust the patient, and we wait a reasonable amount of time to see if the condition resolves itself. But if the headaches don't go away, then, as a health care consumer, the patient needs to say, "Well, I tried this and it helped my spine, but it didn't help the condition I wanted to treat. Now I need to look at another form of care." And as a responsible health care provider, I will absolutely encourage my patients to do so. Headaches can be caused by conditions that are beyond my diagnostic scope (such as a brain tumor). One of the values of conventional medicine is its ability to diagnose a wide range of causes of certain symptoms and offer treatment that may be the only option.

6. **You are the head of your health care team.** No matter what the diagnosis, the patient must make the final decision about any treatment, not the doctor. I believe a doctor, or any other health care provider, is someone that we hire to work for us. He or she is part of our team. The game that this team plays is a serious one: It's life, and our health is the scorecard. It is a game we all want to win for as long as we can.

▶ Using Chiropractic Philosophy as Your Guide to Health

Chiropractic philosophy is probably one of the most sensible and powerful tools you can use to organize your thinking about health and health care. To review some of the basics about chiropractic:

- Chiropractic is the second-largest health care system in the United States. It has been leading the alternative health care movement for more than a hundred years.

- Its philosophy is based on the concept that the same intelligence that animates the universe lies within each human being. The natural expression of this Innate Intelligence is vibrant health and well-being.

- The nerves and nervous system are the conduit through which Innate Intelligence flows from the brain to the body and back again.

- Any impingement on or impediment to the flow of energy and information along the nerves results in a decrease in vitality and thus a decrease in the level of health we experience.

- Chiropractic treats one of the primary sources of nerve impingement, subluxations. These are small misalignments in the bones of the spine that prevent the free flow of information from the brain to the body.

- The chiropractic adjustment is designed to restore the bones of the spine to their full, free range of motion, allowing nerve energy to flow unimpeded once again. When this happens, the body experiences the vibrant health it is designed to have.

Chiropractic philosophy believes that health comes from inside, from the flow of the life force inside us. Chiropractic doesn't wish to add anything to the body, like a drug; instead, it wishes to remove any obstacle to the free flow of Innate Intelligence. It's actually a far more conservative philosophy than 99 percent of conventional medicine!

When you use chiropractic philosophy as your guide to health care choices, it tells you always to use the least invasive method of treatment first. Change your diet instead of taking a pill. Exercise more instead of getting your stomach stapled. Try chiropractic, acupuncture, massage, and physical therapy before you agree to back surgery. Chiropractic philosophy doesn't tell you never to use conventional medicine; there are times when conventional medicine offers the most appropriate treatment option. But chiropractic philosophy can be a valuable guide in areas where your choices aren't so clear-cut. That's when beginning with the least invasive option may be your best health care decision.

The other aspect of chiropractic philosophy that I believe all health care consumers should apply is the importance of patient education. As I said earlier, I believe a doctor's first responsibility is to educate the patient. Chiropractors routinely take time in the first few appointments with new patients to make sure they understand chiropractic philosophy and treatment methods. They also review treatment plans with patients, explaining their recommendations and expected outcomes. After all, educated health care consumers are healthier patients, able to take responsibility for their own health care choices. As a consumer, your responsibility is to seek out the education you need. Do research. Ask questions. Don't automatically rely upon your health care providers to tell you what you need to know. Health care is a partnership, one that works only when both parties are actively involved.

▶ Limitations of Matter

I'll be the first to admit that every philosophy and treatment has its limitations. Any conventional or alternative health care practitioner who tells you otherwise is either naive or deceived. There are philosophic limitations—conventional medical doctors wouldn't diagnose a subluxation even if they saw it because they don't believe in the validity of the concept. There also are limitations produced by training. For instance, an acupuncturist can read your pulse at nine different levels, but he or she might not know what exercises to prescribe for a bad back. Chiropractors' training gives us solid physiological knowledge as well as an understanding of the mechanics of adjustment, but unless we pursue further studies we may not be able to tell you what foods you should eat or what herbs you should take. And an orthopedic surgeon probably can't take very good care of a woman's gynecological issues! Expecting your health care providers to be experts outside their designated specialties is like walking up to a French-speaker and asking him or her to speak Chinese. Each kind of medicine, conventional or alternative, has a body of knowledge in which it is expert, and a much larger body of knowledge in which it isn't. The key is not to expect your health care professional to be an expert in something he or she wasn't trained for. Seek out those practitioners whose knowledge and philosophy are in alignment with your own and are appropriate for your condition and treatment outcomes.

When it comes to the health of the body, however, we run into a much more profound limitation: the limitations of matter. Even though Innate Intelligence underlies every living thing, it expresses itself through matter. There are no limits to Innate Intelligence, but there are limitations to matter.

What does that mean in terms of health care? While chiropractic care helps the body to heal by unblocking the flow of Innate Intelligence, there may be a point where the damage caused by an injury or disease is too extensive for the body's natural ability to heal itself. Say a patient comes to see me because he's been experiencing back pain for years. I take an X ray of the spine, and sure enough, I see degenerative changes that have resulted from years of spinal neglect. One of the disks of the spine has deteriorated to almost nothing. If that patient had sought chiropractic care years ago, I might have been able to prevent the degeneration and save the disk; certainly I can still help this patient by eliminating any subluxations in the spine. But the disk degeneration has gone too far for the body's natural healing ability to save it. This patient may receive enough benefit from chiropractic to reduce or eliminate his pain, but his ability to recover fully is restricted because of the limitations of matter.

Remember another principle of chiropractic: All self-healing occurs through physiological feedback loops. There are local tissue feedback loops, and there are systemic feedback loops generated by the nervous system and the hormonal system. The primary system that facilitates the body's ability to heal is the nervous system. When subluxation interferes with the nervous system, it creates a break in the self-healing feedback loop. Chiropractic is designed to eliminate nerve interference through adjustment of the spine so that the body can heal itself naturally.

When the body is affected by degeneration caused by abnormal repetitive motion, accident, injury, or trauma, in many cases chiropractic can provide extremely effective treatment, marshaling the body's own Innate Intelligence and self-healing ability to take care of the condition. But if degeneration has progressed past the body's ability to heal itself even when the body is free from subluxation, then other methods of treatment may be called upon to restore the body to the greatest degree of health possible. That treatment may include alternative means such as acupuncture, herbs, supplements, massage, physical therapy, homeopathy, psychological support such as hypnosis or therapy, and also conventional medicine.

Even if other healing modalities are used, chiropractic care in many cases can be of enormous support to the body in its healing process. Chiropractors would say that the very first thing you want to do in most illnesses is to make sure the nervous system is free of interference. Many of my patients will come to see me first whenever they become ill. If our treatments don't resolve their condition, then they'll go to their naturopath or acupuncturist or homeopath or medical doctor—whatever other modality that seems appropriate to them or that we decide upon together after discussing their conditions. But usually we also will continue treating them using chiropractic, simply to keep their overall physical health as robust as possible. After all, a body that is in good general health is far more likely to benefit from treatment for specific unresolved conditions.

▶ Taking Charge of Your Health

Being an intelligent health care consumer isn't that hard—but it isn't easy, either. Choices are not always black and white. That's why people often give up their power and say, "Look, you're the doctor. Just do what you need to do." But I believe the best way to take care of your health is to partner with your doctor or health care provider. No one will care for your health more than you do, so you'd better hold up your end of the partnership.

To take responsibility for getting the best health care possible, your job is threefold. First, *ask questions.* The only way you'll understand the treatment being offered to you is to be thorough in your questioning. Doctors of all kinds are experts in their specialties, and they have so much knowledge they may forget that you don't know what they know. So if you don't understand something, ask, and ask again until you get an answer that satisfies you. If you aren't getting satisfactory answers from your doctor, you may want to find another doctor.

Second, *understand the limitations of your health care provider.* Your doctor is not God and can't cure everything. Like every other human being on the planet, you are subject to the limitations of matter. It may not be possible to completely resolve your condition. However, you can expect that your health care provider will do his or her best to restore the maximum amount of health and function possible to your body.

Third, *understand the limitations of your health care provider's philosophy and system of healing.* Doctors want to help and heal people, but they're looking at your condition through the perspective of the way they've been trained. If you go to see a surgeon, what kind of treatment will he or she probably recommend? If you go to a medical doctor, will you likely be prescribed a series of adjustments or a drug? Every doctor is going to want to solve your problem using the tools he or she has. But you, as the patient, are the one who chooses which tools you want used on your body. That begins by choosing the health care providers you wish to consult, and then choosing the treatments you wish to use. As the health care consumer, you need to be able to take a hard look at whatever treatment you're offered and ask, "Am I willing to do this to reach the kind of health I want to achieve? Is this the best way to treat this particular problem?" Ultimately, it means choosing the health care philosophy you feel will offer you the greatest health and vitality.

Each human body is fundamentally the same as other human bodies—and yet infinitely different. The human psyche is even more variable. How you choose to take care of your health depends on both your body and your mind, on the condition of your health and the health care philosophy you feel is closest to your own. There is no approach to health, no health care system, no healing modality that can be all things to all people all the time. Much as we'd like there to be, there is no panacea, no cure that will work for everyone. Every support for your health has its strengths and weaknesses. Your job is to choose what works for you, to insist on getting the information and care you deserve, and to work with your health care providers to gain the greatest benefit from the treatment you receive. When you do so, you can experience joy—not merely the joy of abundant health, but the joy of knowing you have co-created it.

APPENDIX I

Conditions Helped by Chiropractic Care

As I have said, chiropractic's aim is not necessarily to cure disease or even to alleviate symptoms, but to restore the body to optimal functioning by removing blocks to the free flow of Innate Intelligence. Yet most people who seek chiropractic care do so because of their symptoms, usually some sort of pain. Happily, many patients find that a course of chiropractic care does far more than just eliminate the symptoms for which they sought treatment. There are countless case histories of people who have noticed improvements in diseases and conditions afflicting virtually every system in the body. I myself have had patients who reported their emphysema got better, or their eyesight improved, or their blood pressure problems disappeared, or they could get by on lower doses of insulin for their diabetes, or their digestive problems cleared up, and so on.

This appendix is designed to give you an idea of some of the current research findings on how chiropractic care can help heal a wide range of conditions, symptoms, and diseases. Before we look at specific conditions and systems, however, it's important to understand how scientific research is done and how research into the effects of chiropractic care fits into the contemporary scientific method.

▶ Chiropractic Care and Scientific Research

While chiropractic care has been around for over a hundred years, for the first seventy-five of those years research into its effectiveness was based on case studies, reports showing how chiropractic helped one individual overcome a particular health problem. These case studies have been documented and published, but they do not hold the same weight in the scientific community as do controlled double-blind studies.

Controlled double-blind studies are often used when testing drugs on humans. This type of study consists of a control group where people with a certain condition—headaches, for example—are left untreated. Another group of subjects suffering from the same type of headache is given the drug under study to see if it helps to reduce or eliminate their symptoms. A third group is given a placebo (often a sugar pill). Neither the researchers nor the subjects know who is receiving the drug and who is receiving the placebo. Each group is monitored to see if there are changes in their headaches. This kind of study allows researchers to determine if the drug under study has better results than no treatment at all, or better results than the headache relief by those taking the placebo. If the group taking the drug shows significant improvement compared to the control and placebo groups, then the drug is likely to be considered scientifically and clinically useful for treatment of headaches.

It is usually considered better to have a large double-blind study as opposed to a small one because of what is known as sample error or sample bias. We tend to think of science as giving us black-and-white answers, but this is untrue in many cases, especially when studying human beings. Unpredictable responses to drugs or other factors that affect humans can skew the results of tests. (These unpredictable responses are termed "side effects" by the drug companies.) If you are testing only a small number of people—let's say ten—a single individual who responds unpredictably to a drug can throw off the statistics of an entire study. Your study would show that 10 percent of people exhibit the same response to your drug, and such a statistic might be incorrect or biased. However, if you test a larger group—a hundred or a thousand—and the same one person responds unpredictably to your drug but everyone else doesn't, then your results would show a 1 percent (out of 100) or even 0.1 percent (out of 1,000) unpredictable response. According to the scientific method, the larger the group tested, the more likely you are to get statistics that are valid and unskewed by sample error or bias. If you study five people who smoked cigarettes, for example, and they all lived to be ninety-five years old and died of natural causes, you could make the assumption that smoking does not cause any health problems. But if you studied a population of ten thousand smokers and found they had a significantly higher rate of emphysema, lung cancer, and other serious health problems, you would conclude that smoking can cause serious health problems. The size of the study would have a significant impact on the conclusion that is drawn.

Unfortunately, the double-blind method of testing requires large groups of subjects and lots of money. Drug companies traditionally provide the greatest amount of funding for such tests, and their goal, obviously, is to test the efficacy of the drugs they wish to sell. Is it any wonder that there is very little funding for doing double-blind studies of chiropractic care, since it is the most popular form of *drug-free* health care in the United States? Luckily, as the popularity of alternative medicine continues to grow, the numbers of studies in the double-blind category as well as of large population studies in general are increasing. (By the way, scientific studies on the efficacy of alternative medical treatments have been done for many years in Europe and the Far East. Here in the United States we are only just now beginning to recognize these studies as a sound foundation of proof for alternative medicine.)

Research into the scientific basis of chiropractic has taken two different tracks. First is research that validates the fundamental premise of chiropractic—that subluxation of spinal bones interferes with normal physiological function, and this interference manifests itself in a wide variety of health problems. Correction of subluxation restores the full expression of Innate Intelligence (brings the body back to homeostasis). When that occurs, individuals with a wide variety of health problems regain their health. In the References section of this book you'll find citations for a great many studies that have validated the fundamental principles of chiropractic.

The second research track has to do with the effects of chiropractic care on almost every physical condition a human being can present. Up to this point, the majority of such research has taken the form of case studies. (Indeed, the very first report of the effects of chiropractic care was written by chiropractic's founder, D. D. Palmer, who described how a man was cured of deafness with one adjustment.) A case study is by definition a study of a population of one, and some may challenge the validity of such a small sample. But when case study after case study presents the same result, and all those case studies are added together, those numbers strongly support the efficacy of chiropractic care in helping patients to eliminate or alleviate the conditions and diseases listed in this chapter.

I must stress this is not just anecdotal evidence, such as a patient writing down "I feel better!" on a chiropractor's comment form.

Chiropractors are trained medical professionals. They know about the scientific method. They offer very precise treatments to their patients and keep very accurate records of exactly what adjustments were used. They can see for themselves the results of their care, and they are used to quantifying those results by gathering specific information from their patients. Chiropractic journals are filled with precise records of care given and results produced. So when you read the list of symptoms and diseases in this chapter, you can rest assured that the results you see listed have been documented thoroughly with many patients over the decades.

One other point about case studies: They often form the basis for ongoing research. It is not uncommon in medicine to have a person respond unexpectedly to a routine drug or medical treatment. Although the person may be being treated for one condition, the treatment that he or she is getting gives positive results for a seemingly unrelated condition. This scenario (a case study) often leads to further research to determine if the drug or medical procedure can be applied effectively for this other condition. It is unfortunate that while conventional medicine is happy to use its case studies as an indicator for further research, it is far less likely to accept the validity of many years of case studies done in the alternative medical field, which includes chiropractic.

Scientific research into the efficacy of alternative medical care is increasing simply because the public demands it. What you will find below are the results of many years of case studies and other research into the effects of chiropractic. I believe that we will continue to see more and more reports of successful research into both the fundamental principles of chiropractic and specific diseases, symptoms, and conditions that can be helped with chiropractic care. I hope this introduction has given you a clearer understanding of the nature and scope of the research presented in this chapter. This research is only the beginning, but the beginnings are solid enough for you to use as a guide for seeking care for yourself or a loved one.

As you read the different health problems that chiropractic can help, it may seem that I am saying that chiropractic is a cure-all or a panacea. This is not the case. There are usually many causes for any disease state. These causes can range from environmental factors, such as pollution, to diet, trauma, or genetics. What is essentially being proposed here is that correction of subluxation can have a powerful effect on restoring the body toward health. In some cases the chiropractic adjustment may be all that is needed to enable the patient to fully recover from the health problem, while in other cases it may help to improve the condition partly and should be used in conjunction with other modalities. And finally, of course, there are conditions that may have little or no correlation to subluxation.

▶ Conditions That Respond to Chiropractic Care

The following is a list of conditions that have been shown to respond to chiropractic care. Specific diseases are listed alphabetically, as well as different systems of the body. If you have asthma, for instance, you might consult both the entry on asthma and the entry on lung and bronchial problems. In some cases I've noted the specific study or studies that validate chiropractic's effects. If no study is listed, you can check the References section at the back of the book for more information. If a specific condition is discussed elsewhere in this book, you'll find a chapter reference.

The research included here is designed to serve as your guide to a more holistic approach to conditions and diseases. However, these suggestions are not prescriptive. No health practitioner would recommend a course of care unless he or she knew the details of a patient's health. What I do hope this chapter will do is to offer you possible alternative means of treating a condition or augmenting the treatment you are already receiving. And because its focus is on improving the health and function of the entire body, I believe chiropractic care can be of benefit no matter what your condition, and can form a valuable part of any treatment plan.

In compiling this appendix I must acknowledge a huge debt of gratitude to Tedd Koren, D.C. His book *Chiropractic and Spinal Research* (2000 edition) was my primary resource for articles and research. By accumulating thousands of references in one place, he is a tireless contributor to the knowledge base of all chiropractors. I also wish to acknowledge Dr. Malik Slausberg, D.C., who first showed me that more and more people are providing scientific proof of what chiropractors have known all along; the effectiveness of chiropractic in caring for almost every condition found in the human body. Finally, I wish to recognize the major publications in which you will find chiropractic research. They include the *Journal of Chiropractic Research, Journal of Craniomandibular Practice, Journal of Manipulative and Physiological Therapeutics, International Chiropractic Pediatric Association Newsletter, Journal of the American Osteopathic Association, Chiropractic Journal, Chiropractic Pediatrics, Journal of the American Chiropractic Association,* and *Journal of Vertebral Subluxation Research,* as well as journals and publications from England, New Zealand, and Australia.

Allergies. Allergies are caused by a malfunction of the body's natural immune system response. Because chiropractic care restores optimal functioning to the entire body, many patients experience a reduction or elimination of their allergic symptoms. This reduction of symptoms is seen most clearly in children. In one study done at Western States Chiropractic College (1988), 61.6 percent of children with complaints such as ear infections, sinus problems, allergies, bedwetting, and respiratory and gastrointestinal problems received substantial improvement. Another 1973 study indicated that cranial manipulation relieved symptoms of posttraumatic epilepsy, allergic problems, and dizziness in infants and children. See also Chapter 12.

Arthritis. Arthritis takes two common forms, osteoarthritis (age-related degeneration of the joints) and rheumatoid arthritis (an autoimmune disease of collagen, one of the body's primary connective tissues). Interestingly enough, an article published in the *Journal of the American Medical Association* in 1976 noted that rheumatoid arthritis was shown to affect the cervical spine in more than 86 percent of patients with the disease. As a chiropractor, I must ask why would it be true that the cervical area would be involved in so many cases of rheumatoid arthritis. Could it be that subluxations in the cervical area have something to do with triggering the body's abnormal autoimmune response and thus producing the arthritis?

I have discussed using chiropractic in cases of osteoarthritis in Chapter 13. You'll also find some recommendations for supplements for arthritis in Chapter 9.

Asthma. This condition causes more children to be absent from school than any other illness. Luckily, asthma, especially in children, has proven to respond very well to chiropractic care. In one 1997 study of eighty-one children with asthma who were evaluated before and after two months of chiropractic care, 90.1 percent reported less impairment caused by asthma following treatment, and 30.9 percent voluntarily decreased the amount of asthma medication they were taking. Chiropractic care also appeared to decrease the number of asthma attacks by an average of 44.9 percent.

Adults with asthma also appear to improve when they receive regular chiropractic care. In one 1975 study, 95 percent of patients with bronchial asthma reported that both peak flow rate (how much air they could take in) and vital capacity (how much air their lungs could hold at one time) increased after the third visit with their chiropractor.

Attention Deficit Hyperactivity Disorder (ADHD). ADHD is a blanket diagnosis for a range of behavioral and biochemical problems.

Many parents who are concerned about problems with current conventional medical therapy (usually drugs) are seeking healthier, nondrug options for their ADHD children. Luckily, chiropractic care offers hope. While I discuss ADHD in Chapter 12, there are two studies I want to mention here. One, reported in 1980, looked at twenty-four ADHD children, half of whom received stimulant medication such as Ritalin, while the rest received chiropractic care as their only treatment. Those receiving chiropractic care experienced a lessening of hyperactivity and improved attentiveness, as well as improvements in both gross and fine motor coordination. The medicated children also experienced initial improvements in level of hyperactivity and attentiveness, but these improvements decreased over time, requiring higher dosages of drugs to maintain them. There also were no improvements in gross or fine motor coordination in the medicated group. Equally important, over half of the children receiving drugs demonstrated changes in personality, loss of appetite, and insomnia.

In a second, blind study (1989), seven children received chiropractic adjustments and seven others received placebo care. Five of the seven children who were adjusted showed improvement in their levels of hyperactivity. Other case studies demonstrate that many children can be taken off medication and their cases managed completely with chiropractic care.

Autism. There are a number of conditions lumped under the heading of autism, ranging from the mild form now called Asperger's syndrome to disability severe enough to necessitate institutional care. Autistic children exhibit behaviors such as lack of socialization skills, inability to relate to others, and nonverbalization. In its most extreme form autism can produce self-destructive rituals, obsessive-compulsive behaviors, violence, or complete lack of communication with the outside world. There are currently few treatments for autism, although drugs and behavior modification therapy are being used.

Growing case study and anecdotal evidence shows that alternative medicine (chiropractic, nutrition, homeopathy, and so on) can produce good results in many children. In one 1987 study, the authors reported that 50 percent of the autistic children under chiropractic care demonstrated "reliable behavioral improvements, as recorded by independent observers." (The study notes that autism experts consider any change in behavior in an autistic child to be significant.) A recent case study (1999) of a three-and-a-half-year-old girl who was nonverbal, engaged in compulsive behaviors and daily rituals, and exhibited head banging and other violent behavior relates that after one month of chiropractic care her parents and teachers noted a 30 percent improvement in the child's social behavior. In one year, social behavior had improved by 80 percent, and her head banging, rituals, and violent behavior had decreased by 50 percent. If your child is autistic, I suggest a check by a chiropractor for subluxation involvement.

Back pain/sciatica. Back surgery has become the primary treatment offered by conventional medicine for these conditions. It is interesting to note, however, that a 1994 study showed that the rate of back surgery in the United States is 40 percent higher than in any other country, and five times higher than in England or Scotland. It is also unfortunate to note that back surgery all too often fails to resolve the initial complaint of chronic debilitating pain. However, other studies are beginning to show that chiropractic care can provide significant relief in many cases of back pain. In 1999 a study compared the use of spinal manipulation, NSAIDs (nonsterodial anti-inflammatory drugs), and acupuncture on seventy-seven patients with back pain. After thirty days, only patients treated with spinal manipulation showed measurable improvement—50 percent reduction in lower back pain,

46 percent reduction in upper back pain, and 33 percent reduction in neck pain. Acupuncture and NSAIDs produced no significant relief. As another 1999 study stated, "Of the available conservative treatments [for low back pain], chiropractic management has been shown through multiple studies to be safe, clinically effective, cost-effective, and to provide a high degree of patient satisfaction." See Chapter 7 for information about a typical course of chiropractic care for back pain.

Bedwetting. This common childhood ailment has been treated in conventional medicine by behavior modification and drugs with varying levels of success. There is evidence, however, that subluxation can be a contributing factor to bedwetting, and once the subluxations are resolved the condition improves. In a 1991 study of 171 bedwetting children, the average number of incidents was reduced from seven per week to four, and the number of children assessed as "dry" rose from 1 percent to 15.5 percent. Many parents report their children have no bedwetting incidents for several days following chiropractic adjustments.

Behavioral and psychological issues. There are numerous case studies that report positive changes in behavior and psychology in both children and adults following chiropractic care. I want to cite one impressive yet long-forgotten study. For fifteen months in 1930 and 1931, 244 boys who were incarcerated in a reform school in Greendale, Kentucky, were placed under chiropractic care. Of those 244, 155 were considered "completely recovered or greatly benefited" by chiropractic at the end of the fifteen months. Teachers at the school noted improvement in the boys from their first adjustments. Schoolwork, health, and general attitude all improved markedly. The teachers were so impressed, they voluntarily signed a petition asking for a full-time chiropractor for the school. The superintendent of Kentucky's reform schools wrote, "I have been able to notice a marked improvement in the mental and physical condition of the boys and in school work and conduct; also, there has been a larger number of paroles during that period than any previous period during the past four years. . . . We have been able to accomplish results far beyond [our] fondest hopes and expectations in the rehabilitation of these boys." *See also* Emotional health *and* Learning disorders.

Bell's palsy (facial paralysis). Typically a paralysis of one side of the face, Bell's palsy can be caused by trauma to or compression of the nerve or by an "unknown infection" (*Mosby's Medical Dictionary*). Certainly, compression of or trauma to a nerve can involve subluxations. There have been several case studies of children and adults diagnosed with Bell's palsy who have experienced significant improvement and even complete recovery with adjustments. In one such case, reported in October 1997, a five-year-old boy took a fall from his bicycle and over the next week developed symptoms of Bell's palsy—he could not close his right eye or wrinkle his brow. A neurologist told his parents it would probably be four to five months before the child would recover his ability to move his face. However, the parents consulted a chiropractor, who discovered a subluxation in the child's atlas (the bone at the base of the skull). The child received adjustments once a week, and after three weeks he had recovered 90 percent of his facial muscle mobility.

Bladder and urinary tract problems. There are proven links between problems in the lower spine and bladder and urinary tract conditions. One 1988 study reviewed ten case histories, including that of a forty-one-year-old woman with a twenty-year history of bladder, bowel, and gynecological problems. Within two weeks of beginning chiropractic care, her bladder and bowel were functioning normally, and her gynecological problems resolved not long after that. *See also* Pelvic pain *and* Bedwetting.

Brain function. The advent of diagnostic tools such as PET and CAT scans and MRIs, and more advanced knowledge of neuro-transmitters and brain chemistry, have given science much more precise ways to assess the effects of chiropractic care on brain function. One area of study deals with blood flow to the brain and its possible impedance by subluxations and/or blockages in the cervical area of the spine. A 1997 study used PET and SPECT scans to evaluate perfusion and glucose metabolism in the brains of patients with whiplash. (Whiplash patients often report symptoms such as loss of memory and vision and emotional changes, all of which are linked to brain function.) Six whiplash patients and twelve controls were evaluated. The scans of the whiplash patients showed significantly decreased brain function and blood flow to the parietooccipital regions of both the right and left sides of the brain. The study hypothesized that the decrease was due to problems in the nerves of the upper cervical area. *See also* Whiplash.

Breastfeeding difficulties. I regularly see new mothers whose children are having problems breastfeeding. When I interview the mother, I often find there were difficulties in the birth that caused trauma to the child's head and neck. And, as you read in the Introduction and in Chapter 12, after one or two adjustments the child is able to breastfeed successfully. Another cause suggested for breastfeeding difficulties is temporomandibular joint dysfunction (TMJ), again caused by the birth process. In 1993 one thousand newborns who had difficulty nursing were evaluated by a chiropractor, who found that eight hundred of the children, or 80 percent, had some degree of TMJ. More important, when these babies were treated with cranial and spinal adjustments, 99 percent experienced some relief and increased ability to nurse. As I noted in Chapter 12, I recommend all mothers bring their babies in for checkups within two weeks of birth, to make sure any birth-induced subluxations are eliminated.

Breech birth. Breech births (where the baby is born bottom-first instead of headfirst) are far more dangerous for both mother and child, creating the need either for Cesarean rather than vaginal delivery, or for medical intervention to try to turn the child in utero by mechanical means. However, I have found that women receiving regular chiropractic care during their pregnancies are more likely to deliver healthfully and more easily, with the baby presenting headfirst. One chiropractor has developed a specific series of adjustments (the Webster breech technique) that seems to help babies go from breech position to the preferred headfirst presentation.

Bronchitis. *See* Lung and bronchial problems.

Cancer. How can chiropractic, which ostensibly treats the nerves, bones, and muscles, help with cancer? Certainly any care that promotes the overall health and well-being of an individual can be of assistance. I hypothesize that in some cases restoring the flow of Innate Intelligence to its proper levels triggers the body's natural defenses to take up the fight against cancerous cells. There have been case studies as early as the 1940s and as recent as 1998 that recount different kinds of cancer going into remission following chiropractic treatments. The 1998 report describes a sixty-year-old patient with liver cancer who had received medical treatment, gone into remission, and then had the cancer recur. The second remission occurred without further conventional medical treatment while the patient continued his chiropractic care. More important, the report states that "three years [after the remission] the patient is enjoying a life of retirement, and remains under chiropractic care."

The decision to treat cancer through alternative means is

one that must be considered very carefully and made with an awareness of possible consequences. However, I do believe that by restoring greater overall health to the body, alternative medicine—including chiropractic—can be a valuable adjunct in the treatment of cancer, easing side effects, and potentially helping patients heal more quickly.

Cardiovascular health. As early as 1910, D. D. Palmer was reporting a case of a patient with heart trouble whom he examined and in whom he found "a displaced vertebra pressing against the nerves which innervate the heart." After Palmer adjusted the vertebra, the patient experienced "immediate relief." More recent and wider-ranging studies seem to indicate that irritation of the upper thoracic vertebral joints may cause problems with the sympathetic nerves that run to the heart and regulate things like heartbeat rhythm. In one study (1995), eleven patients with heartbeat abnormalities were treated with spinal manipulation, and after one month positive trends were noted in several heart rate factors. For another study (1992), ten chiropractic students volunteered to have their HDL/LDL cholesterol levels monitored for one to three years to assess the possible effects of regular chiropractic care on cardiac risk factors. All ten students had significant reductions in their cardiac risk factors over the course of the study.

Carpal tunnel syndrome. The conventional medical prescription for carpal tunnel syndrome is anti-inflammatory drugs, which are dangerous if taken over the long term, and surgery, which may or may not resolve the problem. However, studies are beginning to demonstrate that chiropractic care, combined with treatments such as ultrasound and wrist supports, is equally as effective without the downside of drug side effects. It is also beginning to be clear that carpal tunnel syndrome often has less to do with the nerves and muscles of the arm and wrist and more to do with the nerves and muscles of the neck and shoulders. In a 1985 study of over a thousand patients, the *Journal of Hand Surgery* noted correlations between carpal tunnel syndrome and cervical arthritis. Rather than undergoing the stress and uncertain outcome of surgery, I suggest my patients try all alternative means at their disposal first—chiropractic, physical therapy, adjustments in their work environment, rest, and so on—to see if their symptoms can be alleviated.

Cerebral palsy. This is still the most prevalent lifelong developmental disability found in the United States. Symptoms include muscle spasticity, intermittent or constant pain, and difficulty with speech. Chiropractic care can be shown to increase the overall health of both children and adults with cerebral palsy. In many cases, the improvement in quality of life is marked. One 1994 study of two children and five adults reported decreases in muscle spasticity, improvement in sleep patterns, decreased pain and irritability, and higher resistance to infections. There was also improvement noted in speech and balance.

Childhood diseases. See Chapter 12; *see also* Colic, Common cold and flu, Ear infections, Fevers, *and* Tonsillitis.

Club foot/hip dysplasia/foot inversion. These disorders of the feet and hips create challenges in walking and standing. They are usually first seen in newborns or very young children, and the standard conventional medical treatment involves splints, casts, and/or surgery. I suggest that children with these conditions be taken to a chiropractor before any medical intervention is done. Sometimes subluxations in specific areas of the spine contribute to such conditions, and reducing the subluxations can ease or eliminate the abnormalities over time. In one such case (1994), a seven-day-old infant had a hip dysplasia that prevented him from extending his left leg. Doctors at the hospital placed the baby in a brace restricting movement of both legs. The parents then took the child to a chiropractor, who diagnosed and treated a sacral subluxation. After that, the child's hip dysplasia disappeared and no further medical treatment was needed.

Colic. A condition where babies cry nonstop, usually because of pain in their digestive tracts. Conventional medical treatment with drugs is only sometimes effective. Chiropractic care offers a healthful, nondrug option to parents. One 1999 randomized controlled trial in Denmark tested two groups of colicky infants. Half received chiropractic care, the other half a drug (dimethicone). Hours the children spent crying were tracked in a diary. By day four, crying had decreased by 1 hour in the medicated babies but had decreased 2.4 hours in the babies receiving chiropractic care. Throughout the trial, chiropractic care proved to be more effective than drugs in reducing crying due to colic. An earlier (1989) study surveyed seventy-three chiropractors who had adjusted 316 infants for moderate to severe colic. Within two weeks of their starting chiropractic care, 94 percent of the children showed improvement, according to their mothers. This improvement was maintained after a period of four weeks. See the Introduction and Chapter 12 for other stories of colicky babies helped by chiropractic care.

Common cold and flu. Many parents find they and their children are much more resistant to infections when they receive regular chiropractic care. In one osteopathic study of over forty-six hundred cases of upper respiratory tract infections, fewer than 5 percent of those patients who were treated with spinal manipulation developed secondary infections or complications—far better results than found in patients treated with drugs.

Constipation. Diet can play a major part in preventing constipation (see Chapter 9). But in many cases, especially with young children, subluxations of specific areas of the spine can prevent the bowel from functioning properly. I frequently see instances of babies and toddlers who haven't had a bowel movement for days experience almost immediate relief after having an adjustment. Regular chiropractic care can help patients establish a more natural rhythm of comfortable, effortless elimination. In some cases patients with irritable bowel syndrome (IBS) who experience constipation also can find resolution of their symptoms with chiropractic care. See also Chapter 12.

Diabetes. There have been instances where diabetics who receive regular chiropractic care have found they could reduce their intake of insulin (1989). Certainly there are several reports of patients noticing improvement in the effects of diabetes. One of the major problems experienced by older diabetics is a loss of feeling in the lower extremities due to circulation problems. This can be serious, as it can lead to injury to or loss of the affected limb. In two separate case studies (1989 and 1994), diabetic patients felt a restoration of warmth and feeling in previously numb feet and legs as a result of chiropractic treatment.

Digestive problems. Difficulties digesting food have reached epidemic proportions in industrialized societies. Approximately 40 percent of adults complain of indigestion or other digestive ailments. While some digestive problems can be managed through dietary choices (see Chapter 9), many patients (statistically around 22 percent) report some improvement in digestive symptoms following visits to their chiropractor. (This makes complete sense when you understand the extensive network of nerves leading to the intestines. Improving nerve function will help the digestive tract to work better.) *See also* Breastfeeding difficulties, Colic, Internal organ disease, *and* Ulcers.

Disk herniation and protrusion. These conditions are the cause of a great deal of chronic and acute back pain suffered by hundreds of thousands of Americans every year. The chiropractic model holds that some cases of disk degeneration can be averted with regular chiropractic care prior to actual degeneration occurring; there are also reports of improvement in both disk herniation and protrusion following chiropractic treatment. A 1996 study described twenty-seven patients with documented disk herniations who were treated with chiropractic adjustments, flexion distraction, physiotherapy, and exercise. MRIs following treatment showed that in 63 percent of patients the disk herniation had either been reduced or completely reabsorbed. Other studies conclude that unless specific conditions that indicate the need for surgery are present, chiropractic is a safe, conservative choice for disk herniation and protrusion. It has also shown to provide a very high degree of patient satisfaction, as it reduces pain and provides greater quality of life for patients. See Chapter 5 and Chapter 7.

Dysmenorrhea (menstrual pain). Several studies have shown that menstrual pain can be reduced using spinal manipulation. Two different studies (one in 1979, another in 1992) demonstrated that women received significant reduction in symptoms of discomfort immediately following adjustments. Blood tests also showed a decrease in levels of prostaglandins. (Prostaglandins are hormonal substances that cause pelvic cramping and muscle spasms, two components of dysmenorrhea.) Control groups (some of whom received sham adjustments, some of whom were monitored only) experienced little or no pain relief.

Ear infections. According to statistics, over 66 percent of children have experienced at least one ear infection (otitis media) by the time they are three years old. The common medical prescription is a course of antibiotics, but there is more and more evidence that indiscriminate usage of such drugs causes more problems than it solves. Most parents would be very happy to find a drug-free solution, and for many children chiropractic care provides just such a solution. Among the many studies and case histories involving ear infections, one large program in 1997 stands out. It involved 332 children, age twenty-seven days to five years, with otitis media that ranged from mild to severe, chronic to acute. All of the children in the study experienced some improvement in their conditions with chiropractic adjustments alone (no antibiotics). It took anywhere from five to six adjustments for the condition to normalize itself over a period of seven to eleven days. The recurrence rate of ear infection was as low as 11 percent when tracked over a six-month period. See also Chapter 12.

Eczema. *See* Skin disorders.

Elimination problems. We seem to be in the middle of an epidemic of digestive and eliminative problems, perhaps in part due to our poor dietary habits. However, chiropractic care can also help resolve many of the conditions and symptoms associated with elimination problems. For example, in a 1995 study, a thirty-one-year-old man with Crohn's disease had not had a normal bowel movement since age fifteen. He suffered from constant abdominal cramps and was on several medications. After a course of chiropractic care, he was able to have normal bowel movements and stop all his medication. See Chapter 9. *See also* Constipation, Digestive problems, *and* Irritable bowel syndrome.

Emotional health. As the conventional medical world begins to accept the idea of mind/body/emotions as one functioning unit, some of the most interesting research being done today focuses on the effects of chiropractic on the brain as well as the body. In particular, studies are being done to quantify what chiropractic patients have reported for years: that they feel more relaxed, calm, and emotionally well-adjusted after a treatment. In one such study (1997) community college students were exposed to a fear-engendering stimulus, creating a phobic reaction, and then muscle-tested to see what spinal segment was linked to the fear response. Next, the students were exposed to the fear stimulus while an adjustment was given to the linked area of the spine. After the adjustment, students were again exposed to the fear stimulus, and they reported a significant decrease in the intensity of the fear they experienced. Another case study describes a fifty-two-year-old woman with chronic panic attacks. She had been taking antidepressants and tranquilizers and receiving counseling and relaxation training, none of which had worked. She began chiropractic care and immediately noticed an improvement. During an attack, her blood pressure was measured at 180/102 and her pulse rate at 120 beats per minute. She had an adjustment and within four minutes her blood pressure had dropped to 140/80 and her pulse to 76. At the time of the report she had been free of panic attacks for two months—"the best she had been in years," according to the study.

Epilepsy/seizure disorders. Epilepsy and other seizures are characterized by "an uncontrolled electrical discharge from the nerve cells of the cerebral cortex" (*Mosby's Medical Dictionary*). They can cause a momentary lapse in consciousness or massive electrical disturbance throughout the body, creating tremors, rigidity, and convulsions. It is theorized that by restoring the healthy connection between the brain and body and bringing balance to the central nervous system (including the brain), chiropractic care can ease or eliminate seizure disorders. Certainly case studies provide some validation for the effectiveness of chiropractic care in such cases. In 1992 EEG tests given both before and after chiropractic adjustments were used to evaluate brain activity in children with seizure disorders. The adjustments reduced so-called negative brainwave activity (which indicated seizures) as measured by the EEGs. More important, over the course of four months the children experienced a reduction in the frequency of seizures.

Patients ranging from very young children to adults have noticed a decrease in the number and severity of their seizures following chiropractic treatment. One fifteen-year-old boy who had had epileptic seizures since birth had been taking at least five antiseizure medications. When he began chiropractic care, the number and frequency of his seizures were reduced markedly. He stopped taking all drugs but one, and the dosage of that drug was cut by two-thirds. Five years later, the boy was still seizure-free while maintaining his chiropractic care and the lower drug intake (1995).

Fevers. Most fevers are part of the body's natural immune response to certain diseases and should be allowed to run their course. With childhood fevers, however, this advice is hard for parents to follow, as a child's fever can spike so high so quickly. If a child is experiencing frequent illnesses and/or fevers, I always recommend that the parents bring the child in for treatment, to make sure there is no subluxation interfering with the body's natural immune system response. In newborns, a condition known as suboccipital strain (usually caused by birth trauma) produces symptoms such as fever, torticollis (see entry), loss of appetite, crying, even swelling of facial tissue and asymmetric development of hips and skull. Suboccipital strain usually can be relieved with one to three chiropractic adjustments, and the child returns to normal.

Fibromyalgia. A form of rheumatism marked by musculoskeletal pain, stiffness, and spasm. Chiropractic care has been shown to alleviate or eliminate most of the prevailing symptoms of the condition. A 1997 study in the *Journal of Manipulative Physiological Therapy* showed that adjustments restore greater range of motion to affected joints while decreasing pain levels and tenderness.

Glaucoma. Defined as elevated pressure inside the eye caused by a buildup of fluid, this condition is most often found in older adults but sometimes in children as well. One case study (1997) involved a seventeen-month-old girl who was brought to the chiropractor by her mother. The girl had had glaucoma since birth and suffered from recurring sinus and eye infections. Prior to treatment, the child's intraocular pressure was measured at 21R and 28L. Following one month of chiropractic care her intraocular pressure had dropped to 17R and 15L. The child was able to go off all medications and maintain normal intraocular pressure levels.

Gynecological issues. Chiropractors often see gynecological issues such as dysmenorrhea, pelvic pain, and so on, linked to problems in the lower back and impairment of the lower sacral nerve root, which can also affect the bladder and bowel. Adjustments to this area can often aid or resolve a wide range of conditions. *See* Dysmenorrhea, Pelvic pain, Infertility, Pregnancy, *and* Menopause.

Head injury. *See* Trauma.

Headache/migraine. These are two of the most common health problems reported by adults in the United States. Upward of 27 percent of those seeking alternative medical care do so for headache. Migraines are a subcategory of headaches and are marked by pain on one side of the head, extreme sensitivity to light, nausea, and other symptoms. Medications may or may not be effective for headache; however, chiropractic has been shown to provide relief in many cases. One 1998 study compared the effectiveness of chiropractic care for migraines with an antidepressant/antianxiety drug, amitriptyline, and with a combination of drug therapy and chiropractic care. Those patients who received chiropractic care alone experienced significant relief on a par with that felt under drug therapy but without the drug's side effects (which include drowsiness, weight gain, dry mouth, as well as increased likelihood of cardiac problems and glaucoma). More important, chiropractic reduced the severity and frequency of headaches as well or better than the other two treatment options. In a separate study (1995), patients who had used drugs and were taken off them started having headaches again, while those treated with chiropractic continued to experience headache relief as well as more energy.

Many people have headaches that are a result of misalignment in the neck and base of the spine. For them, chiropractic can resolve the underlying problem and offer them lasting headache relief. For example, in 1994 twenty-six patients with chronic headaches due to upper cervical joint dysfunction (again, subluxation) were treated using chiropractic. Twenty-four reported a decrease in the severity and frequency of their headaches. Tension headache sufferers also can experience lessening of pain when treated with chiropractic, as recorded in a 1995 study in the *Journal of Manipulation and Physical Therapy*. No matter what the cause of your headache, consult your chiropractor. He or she will probably be able to provide you safe, drug-free relief from pain.

High blood pressure/hypertension. Doctors have known for years that many cases of high blood pressure (also called hypertension) can be managed successfully through diet and exercise rather than medication. But many chiropractors report that adjustments also significantly reduce blood pressure in hypertensive patients. In 1998 a double-blind study of seventy-five patients was done in which one group of patients with elevated blood pressure received adjustments to the thoracic spine area, another group received placebos (movements that seemed to be adjustments but were not), and a third group received no treatment. The adjusted group experienced decreases in both systolic and diastolic blood pressure, while no significant change was noted in either the control or placebo group. Anyone who has experienced high blood pressure should consider adding chiropractic care to his or her treatment regimen of diet and exercise, perhaps even before resorting to blood pressure medication.

Immune system function. Some recent studies suggest the nervous system plays a role in the body's immune response, and since chiropractic care affects the nervous system it may enhance immune function. Much recent research has focused on the effect of chiropractic care on changes in blood chemistry, increases in natural killer cells and antibodies in the blood, response of substance P (see Chapter 4, "Pain and Your Amazing Nervous System"), and other neurotransmitters. One of the most exciting studies in 1994 involved ten HIV-positive patients, five of whom received upper cervical adjustments.

The five patients who were adjusted had a 48 percent increase in CD4 cell counts over a period of six months, indicating an improved immune response. The five patients who were not adjusted had an almost 8 percent *decline* in CD4 levels. See Chapter 12. *See also* Common cold and flu.

Incontinence. *See* Bedwetting *and* Bladder and urinary tract problems.

Indigestion. *See* Digestive problems.

Infertility. Subluxations in the lower spine can have an effect on a woman's fertility. When these subluxations are treated, fertility levels can be heightened, and conception is more likely to occur. Several cases documented in the 1990s describe women who became pregnant after a course of chiropractic care. One patient, age thirty-two, hadn't menstruated for twelve years yet had been trying to get pregnant using fertility pills and shots prescribed by her medical doctor. After two months of chiropractic adjustments (specifically in the lumbar area), she had her first period, and four months later she conceived. When she went back to her conventional medical doctor, he told her she couldn't be pregnant since he had done everything medically possible to help her and nothing had worked. The patient had a healthy son several months later.

Internal organ disease. As early as 1921, Henry Winsor (a medical doctor) decided to see if there was any correlation between diseased organs, the nerves connected to them, and the vertebrae associated with those nerves. He performed autopsies of seventy-five human bodies and twenty-two cats. He found nearly a 100 percent correlation between "minor curvatures" of the spine and diseases of internal organs. A later (1968) radiography study by an osteopathic physician showed that many patients with various internal organ diseases (gallbladder, stomach, pancreas, etc.) had some displacement of specific areas of the spine. Nowadays it is theorized that displacement of the spine can affect both the parasympathetic and sympathetic nervous systems, causing a wide range of symptoms and organic conditions, including diseases of the internal organs. It makes sense, therefore, that treating related areas of the spine can produce relief of symptoms or, in some cases, alleviation of problems with internal organs. For instance, one patient who was diagnosed medically with crystals in his gallbladder (a pre-gallstone condition) received an adjustment and noticed his gallbladder felt inflamed for the next two weeks. However, when he returned to his conventional medical doctor, he was told all the crystals were now gone. The patient said later he believed the feeling of inflammation was a "curative response" (1921). *See also* Bladder and urinary tract problems, Cancer, Cardiovascular health, Digestive problems, Elimination problems, Gynecological issues, High blood pressure/hypertension, Infertility, *and* Lung and bronchial problems.

Interstitial cystitis. A serious condition of the bladder where cysts form inside, causing pain during urination and scarring. In 1991 the *British Journal of Neurology* published a study in which a link was found between interstitial cystitis and compression of the dorsal nerve root. When the nerve was released (in this case through surgery), the patients experienced immediate relief of pain and other symptoms. Anecdotal evidence among chiropractors indicates adjustments in the same area provide good results as well.

Irritable bowel syndrome (IBS). A chronic disorder affecting 15 to 25 percent of adults, IBS causes cramping, abdominal pain, diarrhea or constipation, and heartburn. Chiropractic care has been shown to help digestive and elimination problems, and it is also effective in cases of IBS (without the side effects of conventional medical drug therapy). One young woman had been afflicted with IBS symptoms once or twice a week for five years. After one session of chiropractic she noticed an easing of symptoms, and within a short time all her digestive problems disappeared. Two years later she was still symptom-free (1996).

Knee problems. Pain and loss of function in the knee joint are often a result of either traumatic injury or long-term improper joint mechanics. In these cases, often there are problems with the spine that may be contributing to the malfunction of the knees. Treating problems in the spine, therefore, can produce a resolution of the knee condition. In one case study (1993), a thirty-five-year-old man who had suffered from chronic knee pain for fifteen years went for chiropractic care, which resolved the condition. Then the man had a car accident and was diagnosed with whiplash. At the same time, his knee began to swell and he experienced severe pain. After another series of adjustments, however, the man's knee was restored to normal function and the pain disappeared.

Learning disorders. The diagnosis of learning disorder can have multiple components—sensory or motor skill impairment, decreased or inappropriate brain function, ADHD (see entry), behavioral issues, and so on. As early as 1975 researchers were studying children diagnosed with learning disorders who received chiropractic care. In many cases, students showed marked improvement in most if not all of the areas where they had been experiencing difficulties. A few examples: A high school student had been failing three subjects and demonstrating multiple discipline, morale, and coordination problems. After undergoing a course of chiropractic care he passed all his subjects, was able to join in athletics, and discontinued all medication. A junior high student who had been hyperkinetic from birth with indications of neurological problems was only passing two subjects, even though he tested at above-average intelligence levels. After chiropractic care, his motor skills improved to the point where he played on a championship Little League team, was promoted with his grade, and made excellent academic progress the following year. An elementary school student was diagnosed as either brain-damaged or retarded, and also suffered from severe emotional problems. Once he started chiropractic care, however, his self-confidence improved to the point where he took part in public speaking activities at his school. His cognitive abilities were retested and showed he was of normal intelligence for his age and grade level. In another 1986 study of children with learning disabilities being treated by chiropractic, significant improvements were noted in visual perception and short-term memory, as well as motivation, attitude, and performance in school. The children also demonstrated measurable increases in IQ scores (8 points full scale, 12 points performance scale). See also Chapter 12.

Lung and bronchial problems. Since the lungs are connected to the spine by an extensive network of nerves, it's not surprising that chiropractic can have a dramatic effect on the health of the respiratory system. In cases where there is diagnosed abnormality in respiratory function, chiropractic care has been shown to bring patients to a greater degree of normal functioning, increasing both airflow and lung capacity (1975). Chiropractic care can also help those with diseases of the lungs and bronchi (pneumonia, bronchitis, etc.) to heal more quickly.

Menopause. While menopause is a natural stage in a woman's life, the symptoms (including hot flashes, night sweats, vaginal dryness, depression, joint pain, and fatigue) can be difficult to endure. In one 1994 osteopathic study, fifteen of thirty patients with menopausal symptoms received manipulative therapy and fifteen received placebo treatment. The group who received therapy experienced a significant drop in symptoms compared with the control group. Other case studies indicate chiropractic and osteopathic care can help make the change of life easier and more healthful for women.

Multiple sclerosis (MS). A progressive disease of the nervous system in which the patient gradually loses the myelin sheath around the nerves, resulting in muscle weakness, stiffness, tingling, loss of balance, and sensory disturbances. There is currently no conventional medical cure and very little help offered for MS patients. However, there are documented cases (from 1945 to the present day) of patients with MS responding favorably to chiropractic care. In several such cases, symptoms were reduced or disappeared altogether, and patients were able to live normal lives. Since chiropractic care helps restore the health of the central nervous system, it makes sense that MS would respond to such alternative means.

Muscular dystrophy (MD). MD involves the degeneration of muscles for no apparent reason (although there is some indication genetics may be a factor). The only treatments offered by conventional medicine are physical therapy and orthopedic surgery "to minimize deformity" (*Mosby's Medical Dictionary*). Fortunately, chiropractic care can also be used to support patients with MD. In 1994 a study of some seventy individuals with Duchenne's muscular dystrophy demonstrated that chiropractic helped to slow the degeneration of muscles created by the condition.

Musculoskeletal conditions (bones, joints, muscles, etc.). Since chiropractic care is intimately involved with the musculoskeletal systems of the body, almost any systemic affliction of the muscles, bones, or soft tissues can often be eased and/or eliminated with chiropractic treatment. In addition, if the problem is with one of the extremities—a foot, hand, arm, or leg, for example—often there is some corresponding subluxation in the spine. The subluxation either caused the problem or, in the case of accident, may have been created at the same time. If you go to a conventional medical doctor and are diagnosed with a musculoskeletal problem, a visit to your chiropractor will certainly do no harm and may help resolve your condition quickly and without drugs or surgery. See Chapters 4 and 5 for more information on the basics of chiropractic care.

Myasthenia gravis. This condition produces muscle weakness, especially in the face and throat. It eventually can affect the muscles involved in respiration. The conventional medical treatment of choice is an anticholinesterase, but use of these drugs over time can be toxic. Case studies of both children and adults have shown significant relief from symptoms and improvement of functioning following chiropractic care. In the case of a sixty-three-year-old man, he was able to discontinue medication and resume a normal life (1999).

Neck pain. *See* Back pain/sciatica *and* Whiplash.

Nervous system disorders and neurological development in children. As noted in a 1992 study, children with neurological problems of many different kinds experience relief and improvement in both sensory and motor functions following chiropractic treatment. One boy's care and development was followed over the course of eight years of chiropractic care and other alternative health care approaches. The child was first brought to the chiropractor at age twenty-two months. He had been diagnosed with spinal meningitis, cerebral palsy, physical and mental retardation, seizures, and a range of other sensory and motor problems. Conventional medicine had provided no solutions other than antiseizure medication. Over the course of his chiropractic care, however, the boy became fully ambulatory and was able to interact with children his own age as well as adults. In 1994, the study reported he was mainstreamed successfully into his own age group at a regular public school.

Pelvic pain. Pelvic pain and organic dysfunction (PPOD) is diagnosed in thousands of women every year. Many women who receive chiropractic adjustments in the pelvic area find their pain and other problems resolve within a very short amount of time. In one case (1990), a woman had experienced eighteen years of pelvic pain and undergone a horrific list of surgical treatments (appendectomy, partial hysterectomy, removal of her left ovary, three exploratory bowel surgeries for her continuous diarrhea, and four bladder surgeries), none of which helped. She came to chiropractic care complaining of sexual dysfunction (inability to experience orgasm) and constant pain. Within eight weeks of starting chiropractic her pain was gone, her diarrhea had vanished, and her other symptoms had lessened. After thirty weeks of chiropractic care she also attained the ability to have an orgasm.

Pregnancy. Up to 90 percent of women experience some kind of back and spinal problems during pregnancy (not surprising, since a woman's body must accommodate the constantly shifting volume of the uterus, which presses on the organs and nerves of the trunk). Because most drug-based treatments can have negative effects on the fetus, chiropractic care provides an excellent drug-free option for elimination of pain and promotion of the mother's health. In 1987 the American Medical Association released records showing that women who received chiropractic care during the third trimester of pregnancy were able to carry their babies to term and deliver them in greater comfort. The need for painkillers during delivery also was reduced by half. Other studies indicate that women who receive regular chiropractic care during pregnancy have shorter and easier labors. See Chapter 12.

Premenstrual syndrome (PMS). PMS can consist of both physical and psychological symptoms, including lower back pain, abdominal bloating, breast tenderness, mood swings, tension, irritability, depression, change in eating habits, variations in sex drive, and cognitive impairment. Several studies have shown that chiropractic care can ease or eliminate most if not all of these symptoms. One 1992 study reported improvements of 44 to 70 percent in psychological factors, while other case studies show complete reversal of physical difficulties caused by PMS. (An Australian study of fifty-four women diagnosed with PMS revealed that PMS sufferers were more likely to have spinal dysfunction—cervical, thoracic, and lower back tenderness and weakness—than a control group.)

Psoriasis. *See* Skin disorders.

Respiratory ailments. *See* Lung and bronchial problems.

Scoliosis. See Chapter 12.

Sexual function. Several studies have indicated that injury or pain in the lumbar spine area can result in sexual dysfunction both in men and in women. Relieving subluxations in this area can restore function by taking pressure off the nerves that run to the sexual organs. *See also* Gynecological issues, Pelvic pain, *and* Back pain/sciatica.

Sudden infant death syndrome (SIDS). See Chapter 12.

Sinus and sinusitis. Cervical subluxations, especially of the atlas, can be a contributing factor in sinus problems and infections (sinusitis), especially in children. If you find a child is prone to infections of the ear, sinuses, or tonsils, have your chiropractor check the child and adjust as needed. See also Chapter 12.

Skin disorders. You wouldn't think that adjustments would have much of an effect on skin diseases, but certainly restoring the overall health of the body cannot help but improve the state of the body's largest organ: the skin. Other alternative medical remedies, such as changes in diet, herbal preparations, stress reduction, acupuncture, and so on, may be used. In cases of psoriasis and eczema, a combination of chiropractic care, careful dietary monitoring, and other natural remedies may be as effective, if not more so, than the current conventional medical drug-based recommendations.

Sleep disorders. Sleep disruptions can be created by a wide range of causes, but often there is underlying pain or disturbance of the body's normal state of homeostasis. Restoring the body to balance allows it to fall asleep naturally. One of the clearest examples of this is in newborns and toddlers. As every parent will tell you, if a newborn's sleep patterns are disrupted, no one sleeps! There have been numerous studies done on the effects of chiropractic care on children's sleep patterns. As you read in Chapter 12, many children (possibly as many as 75 percent) come into this world experiencing some kind of spinal trauma during birth. Eliminating the subluxations created by birth trauma usually creates a deep relaxation in these tiny patients, resulting in more restful sleep for them and their parents. Similarly, many of my patients report improvement in their sleep habits as well as the quality of sleep (how rested they feel) following a course of chiropractic adjustments.

Stuttering. While stuttering can be the result of a number of physical, behavioral, and emotional components, it can also be an indication of an impediment in the pathway from the brain to the nerves and muscles of the mouth. Some children will begin stuttering after a fall or some other neuromusculoskeletal trauma. By eliminating subluxation blocks to the clear communication of information from the brain to the body, chiropractic care can help ease stuttering behavior in some cases. One such case was reported in 1994, in which a seven-year-old boy who presented with stuttering, learning difficulties, hyperactivity, and one leg shorter than the other underwent two months of thrice-weekly adjustments. By the eighth visit, his legs balanced for the first time, his hyperactivity had vanished, and he had stopped stuttering.

Temporomandibular joint (TMJ) syndrome. The temporomandibular joint connects the jawbone to the temporal bone of the skull. TMJ syndrome is a condition in which the joint causes pain or does not function properly. TMJ syndrome is usually treated by dentists and oral surgeons, but because the placement of head, neck, and jaw are intricately linked, chiropractic care can help alleviate any cranial or cervical subluxations that may be contributing to the condition. One 1995 case history described an incidence where a dentist and a chiropractor worked together on a TMJ syndrome patient. As the mandibular position changed, the chiropractic adjustments helped the patient's head and neck accept and hold the new jaw position.

Thyroid. Hypothyroidism (not enough thyroid activity) and hyperthyroidism (too much activity) can affect the body's entire endocrine system. There have been some links established between abnormal thyroid levels and subluxations within the cervical area. Adjustments of these cervical subluxations can improve thyroid function. One young woman with hyperthyroidism had been on medication for six years. She stopped medication and began chiropractic care, and within four months her thyroid levels were normal and her symptoms disappeared (1989).

Tinnitus. Ringing in the ears is another neurological problem for which conventional medicine has few answers. Spinal and cranial manipulation can offer help in some cases, especially if the tinnitus has produced neck and jaw tension. In one case a woman with tinnitus experienced a 50 percent reduction in intensity. She also felt less tense, and her sleep (which had been severely disrupted) improved. A recent study showed that correction of upper neck subluxation resulted in the complete elimination of tinnitus symptoms in nine out of nine cases.

Tonsillitis. In 1989 a survey was taken of two hundred pediatricians and two hundred chiropractors selected at random. They were asked questions about the health of their own children to determine if there were any differences based on chiropractic versus conventional health care models. Almost 43 percent of pediatricians' children had had tonsillitis, compared to under 27 percent of chiropractors' children. Another 1991 study conducted in England showed that when twenty-seven children were treated for tonsillitis with spinal manipulation, symptoms completely disappeared in twenty-five of them. Chiropractors theorize that subluxations in the cranial and cervical areas contribute to a child's tendency to infections of the head and throat areas.

Torticollis. A condition where the neck is twisted to one side, often appearing in children at birth (it's estimated that up to 2 percent of infants have congenital torticollis). Conventional medical treatment includes surgery on the neck muscles and tendons, physical therapy, and in some cases drugs. Luckily, torticollis responds extremely well to chiropractic intervention, usually a combination of spinal adjustment, cranial work, and soft-tissue therapy. When working with such young children, the amount of force used is gentle, and the results often are remarkable. One case history (1998) describes a seven-month-old with congenital muscular torticollis who had undergone several weeks of physical therapy without success. After six sessions of chiropractic care (low-force adjustments and myofascial release work), the torticollis disappeared. One year later the child showed no trace of torticollis.

Tourette's syndrome. A neuropsychiatric condition thought to be caused by chemical imbalances in the brain. Tourette's patients exhibit tics, inappropriate vocalizations, and intermittent involuntary movements. While case studies of patients with Tourette's receiving chiropractic care are few, one child whose Tourette's was diagnosed a month after a head injury experienced a noticeable change in symptoms within three weeks and was asymptomatic most of the time after four months (1998).

Trauma. I am defining trauma here as injury to the body caused by violent movement (sports injury, automobile accident, falls, etc.). While conventional medicine provides very valuable treatment in cases of trauma, there is often residual injury to the spine, neck, and head that trauma doctors may not see. Unfortunately, such injuries may have long-term physical and cognitive effects. In one 1995 study, seventy-eight young children who had gone to the hospital with mild head injuries (upon evaluation, the injuries were not considered severe enough to require hospital admission) were compared with eighty-six children who had sustained minor injury in another area of the body. Both groups were evaluated for cognitive performance in the year following the accident and again at age six and a half. The children with head injuries scored lower on cognitive tests both at the one-year mark and later. They were also more likely to have needed help with reading.

Chiropractic care has been shown to ameliorate the effects of trauma in both children and adults. Even in cases of paralysis following accident, chiropractic adjustments have helped restore certain levels of functionality. One 1993 case of an eleven-year-old boy who had lost the use of his arms and legs following a high-jump accident reported that the child experienced almost full functionality after three months of chiropractic care. Prior to that time, he had not responded to three months of hospital care, including steroid therapy. Following any kind of trauma it is very important to have yourself checked by a chiropractor to make sure that subluxation-based damage to the spine and neck is treated promptly. See Chapter 12.

Ulcers. While antibacterial drugs have become the treatment of choice for ulcers, there is evidence that spinal manipulation can help in the healing process. In 1993 a study was done of adults with duodenal ulcers. Sixteen received chiropractic care, while forty others received conventional medical treatment. The patients who were treated with chiropractic reported pain relief and healing after one to nine days, with the average healing time of 3.8 days. The patients treated with conventional medicine took ten days longer to report healing. *See also* Internal organ disease.

Vertigo. The loss of balance and one's sense of orientation in space, vertigo is often accompanied by headache, nausea, or neck pain. The condition is often attributed to problems with the inner ear. However, there are several reports of vertigo being reduced or eliminated with adjustments to the upper cervical area of the spine. In 1995 a seventy-one-year-old woman who had experienced sudden-onset severe disabling vertigo had sought medical treatment for a year with no relief. She received cervical adjustments that completely resolved the condition. See also Chapter 14 for a story of a patient of mine who suffered from vertigo.

Vision problems. It is not uncommon for chiropractic patients to report improvements in their vision (see Dan's story in the Introduction, and Mildred's story in Chapter 13). Any kind of head trauma or impingement on the nerves that run to the eyes, or the muscles that surround the eyes, can have a dramatic effect on our sight. Chiropractic adjustments, especially those of the upper cervical area, seem to improve visual acuity in patients of all ages and help with conditions such as blurred vision, contraction of visual field, spots before the eyes, eye muscle dysfunction, dry or tearing eye, and so on. Interestingly, some patients whose vision was rated as normal before their treatment noticed an increase in visual sensitivity afterward (1996).

Whiplash. Whiplash is an injury to the neck (the cervical vertebrae and their supporting ligaments and muscles), usually caused by traumatic events such as rear-end car collisions. Patients with whiplash may continue to have problems for years following the trauma that caused the injury. However, many of the problems don't show up on X rays or EKGs but are experienced as ongoing neck pain, back pain, headaches, dizziness, and even neurological or perceptual difficulties. Current conventional medical treatments (drugs, surgery, occasionally physical therapy) may at times relieve symptoms but do nothing to help the cause. Chiropractors believe that much of the trauma of whiplash is due to subluxations and soft-tissue damage created by violent movement experienced in the neck and spine. Regular adjustments can help the body return to its proper positioning and functioning, giving the soft tissues a chance to heal and the nerves to restore their pathways. Some studies indicate that in whiplash cases, the more adjustments the patient receives per week the shorter the duration of care needed to restore the body to proper functioning.

The research in this appendix just scratches the surface of what is available, should you wish to explore further. But most people aren't interested in how much research is available; all they want to know is whether chiropractic can help them or their child or their parents. The bottom line is that chiropractic can provide help for many conditions simply by restoring the body to the highest level of functioning possible. And chiropractic can almost always increase what most people consider of primary importance: quality of life. Surveys in the United States, New Zealand, Canada, Australia, England, Italy, Germany, and many other countries show that chiropractic patients rate themselves highly in physical function, lack of pain, overall health and wellness, energy and vitality, mental health and acuity, and social interactions. So no matter what your condition or state of health, I encourage you to make the choice to incorporate chiropractic care as a support for your life.

APPENDIX II

Chiropractic Colleges
in the United States and Canada

► Chiropractic Colleges in the United States

Cleveland Chiropractic College—Kansas City
6401 Rockhill Road
Kansas City, MO 64131
(800) 467-2252 • (816) 501-0100
www.clevelandchiropractic.edu

Cleveland Chiropractic College—Los Angeles
590 North Vermont Avenue
Los Angeles, CA 90004
(800) 466-2252 • (323) 660-6166
www.clevelandchiropractic.edu

Life Chiropractic College
1269 Barclay Circle
Marietta, GA 30060
(800) 543-3202 • (770) 426-2884
www.life.edu

Life Chiropractic College West
25001 Industrial Boulevard
Hayward, CA 94545
(800) 788-4476 • (510) 780-4500
www.lifewest.edu

Logan College of Chiropractic
1851 Schoettler Road
P.O. Box 1065
Chesterfield, MO 63006
(800) 782-3344 • (636) 227-2100
www.logan.edu

National University of Health Sciences
(formerly National College of Chiropractic)
200 E. Roosevelt Road
Lombard, IL 60148
(800) 826-6285 • (630) 629-2000
www.nuhs.edu

New York Chiropractic College
2360 State Route 89
P.O. Box 800
Seneca Falls, NY 13148
(800) 234-6922
www.nycc.edu

Northwestern Health Sciences University
2501 West 84th Street
Bloomington, MN 55431-1599
(800) 888-4777
www.nwhealth.edu

Palmer College of Chiropractic
1000 Brady Street
Davenport, IA 52803
(800) 722-3648 • (563) 884-5656
www.palmer.edu

Palmer College of Chiropractic West
90 E. Tasman Drive
San Jose, CA 95134
(866) 303-7939 • (408) 944-6000
www.palmer.edu

Palmer College of Chiropractic Florida
4705 Clyde Morris Boulevard
Port Orange, FL 32129
(866) 585-9677
www.palmer.edu

Parker College of Chiropractic
2500 Walnut Hill Lane
Dallas, TX 75229-5668
(800) 438-6932
www.parkercc.edu

Sherman College of Straight Chiropractic
2020 Springfield Road
P.O. Box 1452
Spartanburg, SC 29304
(800) 849-8771
www.sherman.edu

Southern California University of Health Sciences
(formerly Los Angeles College of Chiropractic)
16200 E. Amber Valley Drive
Whittier, CA 90609
(800) 221-5222 • (562) 902-3330
www.scuhs.edu

Texas Chiropractic College
5912 Spencer Highway
Pasadena, TX 77505
(800) 468-6839 • (281) 487-1170
www.txchiro.edu

University of Bridgeport College of Chiropractic
75 Linden Avenue
Bridgeport, CT 06601
(888) 822-4476
www.bridgeport.edu

Western States Chiropractic College
2900 N.E. 132nd Avenue
Portland, OR 97230
(800) 641-5641 • (503) 256-3180
www.wschiro.edu

▶ Chiropractic Colleges in Canada

Canadian Memorial Chiropractic College
1900 Bayview Avenue
Toronto, Ontario
Canada M4G 3E6
(416) 482-2340
www.cmcc.ca

Université du Québec Trois-Rivières Chiropractic Program
3351, Boulevard des Forges
C.P. 500
Trois-Rivières, Québec
Canada G9A 5H7
(819) 376-5011
www.uqtr.ca

REFERENCES

Allen, J.M. 1993. The effects of chiropractic on the immune system: a review of the literature. *Chiropractic Journal of Australia* 23:132–35.

American Medical Association. 1987. AMA study shows that pregnant women under chiropractic care have easier pregnancy and delivery. American Medical Association records released during trial in U.S. District Court Northern Illinois Eastern Division, No. 76C 3777.

Arcadi, V.C. 1993. Birth induced TMJ dysfunction: the most common cause of breast-feeding difficulties. *Proceedings of the National Conference on Chiropractic and Pediatrics, October 1993, Palm Springs, CA.* Arlington, VA: International Chiropractors Association.

Atkins, R.C., M.D. 2002. *Dr. Atkins' New Diet Revolution.* New York: Avon.

Benson, H., M.D., with M. Stark. 1996. *Timeless Healing: The Power and Biology of Belief.* New York: Simon & Schuster.

Berkson, D.L. 1991. Osteoarthritis, chiropractic, and nutrition: osteoarthritis considered as a natural part of a three stage subluxation complex: its reversibility; its relevance and treatability by chiropractic and nutritional correlates. *Medical Hypotheses* 36(4):356–67.

Biedermann, H.J. 1992. Kinematic imbalances due to suboccipital strain in newborns. *Manual Medicine* 6:151–56.

Bloomquist, Michele. 2001. The all meat diet: do today's carnivorous, low-carbohydrate diet plans really work? *WebMD Medical News,* Jan. 1. http://www.webmd.com.

Blum, C.L. 1998. Spinal/cranial manipulative therapy and tinnitus: a case history. *Chiropractic Technique* 10:163–68.

Blunt, K.L., M.H. Rajwani, and R.C. Guerriero. 1997. The effectiveness of chiropractic management of fibromyalgia patients: a pilot study. *Journal of Manipulative and Physiological Therapeutics* 20(6):389–99.

Boline, P.D., K. Kasaak, G. Bronfort, C. Nelson, and A.V. Anderson. 1995. Spinal manipulation versus amitriptyline for the treatment of chronic tension-type headaches: a randomized clinical trial. *Journal of Manipulative and Physiological Therapeutics* 18:148–54.

Braslavsky, Andrea M., M.S. 1999. Protein is the darling of the dieting set—for now. High-protein diets offer fast weight loss and potential problems. *WebMD Medical News,* Nov. 25. http://www.webmd.com.

Brennan, P.C., D.C. Kokjohn, C.L. Kaltinger, et al. 1991. Enhanced phagocytic cell respiratory burst induced by spinal manipulation: potential role of substance P. *Journal of Manipulative and Physiological Therapeutics* 14(7):399–408.

Brennan, P.C., J.J. Triano, M. McGregor, et al. 1992. Enhanced neutrophil respiratory burst as a biological marker for manipulation forces: duration of the effect and association with substance P and tumor necrosis factor. *Journal of Manipulative and Physiological Therapeutics* 15(2):83–89.

Brennan, T.A., L.L. Leape, N.M. Laird, L. Hebert, A.R. Localio, A.G. Lawthers, J.P. Newhouse, P.C. Weiler, and H.H. Hiatt. 1991. Incidence of adverse events and negligence in hospitalized patients. Results of the Harvard Medical Practice Study I (abstract). *New England Journal of Medicine* 324:377–84. http://www.nejm.org.

Brown, M., and P. Vaillancourt. 1993. Case report: upper cervical adjusting for knee pain. *Chiropractic Research Journal* 2(3).

Browning, J.E. 1988. Chiropractic distractive decompression in the treatment of pelvic pain and organic dysfunction in patients with evidence of lower sacral nerve root compression. *Journal of Manipulative and Physiological Therapeutics* 11(5):426–32.

————. 1990. Mechanically induced pelvic pain and organic dysfunction in a patient without low back pain. *Journal of Manipulative and Physiological Therapeutics* 13:406–11.

————. 1995. Distractive manipulation protocols in treating the mechanically induced pelvic pain and organic dysfunction patient. *Chiropractic Technique* 7:1–11.

————. 1996. The mechanically induced pelvic pain and organic dysfunction syndrome: an often-overlooked cause of bladder, bowel, gynecological, and sexual dysfunction. *Journal of the Neuromusculoskeletal System* 4:52–66.

Bryner, P., and P.G. Staerker. 1996. Indigestion and heartburn: a description study of prevalence in persons seeking care from chiropractors. *Journal of Manipulative and Physiological Therapeutics* 19(5):317–23.

Brzozowske, W.T., and E.V. Walton. 1980. The effect of chiropractic treatment on students with learning and behavioral impairments resulting from neurological dysfunction (parts 1 and 2). *Journal of Australian Chiropractic Association* 11(7):13–18 and (8):11–17.

Burchett, G.D. 1968. Segmental spinal osteophytosis in visceral disease. *Journal of the American Osteopathic Association* 67(6):675.

Burnier, A. 1995. The side effects of chiropractic adjustment. *Chiropractic Pediatrics* 1(4).

Cagle, P. 1995. Cervicogenic vertigo and chiropractic, managing a single case—a case report. *Journal of the American Chiropractic Association* (May):83–84.

Capra, F. 1975. *The Tao of Physics.* Boston: Shambhala Publications.

———. 1982. *The Turning Point.* New York: Simon & Schuster.

Cherkin, D.C., R.A. Deyo, J.D. Loeser, T. Bush, and G. Waddell. 1994. An international comparison of back surgery rates. *Spine* 19(11):1201–6.

Childs, N., S. Freerksen, and A. Plourde. 1992. The impact of chiropractic care on established cardiac risk factors: a case study. *Chiropractic: The Journal of Chiropractic Research and Clinical Investigation* 8(2).

Chinappi, A.S., Jr., and H. Getzoff. 1995. The dental-chiropractic co-treatment of structural disorders of the jaw and temporomandibular joint dysfunction. *Journal of Manipulative and Physiological Therapeutics* 18(7):476–78.

Chopra, D., M.D. 1989. *Quantum Healing: Exploring the Frontiers of Mind/Body Medicine.* New York: Bantam Books.

———. 1993. *Ageless Body, Timeless Mind: The Quantum Alternative to Growing Old.* New York: Harmony Books.

Cleary, C., and J.P. Fox. 1994. Menopausal symptoms: an osteopathic investigation. *Complementary Therapies in Medicine* 2:181–86.

Clendening, L., M.D., compiler. 1942. *Source Book of Medical History.* New York: Dover Publications.

Cleveland Clinic. 1999. Understanding arthritis. *Health Topics A–Z.* http://www.webmd.com.

Colin, N. 1998. Congenital muscular torticollis: a review, case study, and proposed protocol for chiropractic management. *Topics in Clinical Chiropractic* 5(3):27–33.

Collins, K.F., et al. 1994. The efficacy of upper cervical chiropractic care on children and adults with cerebral palsy: a preliminary report. *Chiropractic Pediatrics* 1(1):13–15.

Conway, C.M. 1997. Chiropractic care of a pediatric glaucoma patient: a case study. *Journal of Clinical Chiropractic Pediatrics* 2 (2).

Coulter, I.D., et al. 1996. Chiropractic patients in a comprehensive home-based geriatric assessment, follow-up and home promotion program. *Topics in Clinical Chiropractic* 3(2):46–55.

Courtouise, J. 2001. Medicine in the year 1000. *World Book Online,* http://www.worldbookonline.com. Chicago, IL: World Book, Inc.

Crystal, R. 1997. ADD, enuresis, toe walking. *International Chiropractic Pediatric Association Newsletter* (May/June).

Davis, Jeanie. 2002. Medication errors rampant in hospitals but changes are under way to ensure accuracy, safety. *WebMD Medical News,* Sept. 10. http://www.webmd.com.

Davis, P.T., J.R. Hulbert, K.M. Kassak, et al. 1998. Comparative efficacy of conservative medical and chiropractic treatments for carpal tunnel syndrome: a randomized clinical trial. *Journal of Manipulative and Physiological Therapeutics* 21(5):317–26.

DeNoon, Daniel. 2002. Hospital drug-error trends continue: new report finds old problems, but a willingness to change. *WebMD Medical News,* May 24. http://www.webmd.com.

Doheny, Katherine. 2000. Food for your blood? *WebMD Medical News,* Jul. 24. http://www.webmd.com.

Dusky, Lorraine. 2002. The Atkins diet. *Food and Nutrition,* WebMD, Inc. http://www.webmd.com.

————. 2002. The Pritikin principle. *Food and Nutrition,* WebMD, Inc. http://www.webmd.com.

————. 2002. The Zone diet. *Food and Nutrition,* WebMD, Inc. http://www.webmd.com.

Eliyahu, D.J. 1996. Magnetic resonance imaging and clinical follow-up: study of 27 patients receiving chiropractic care for cervical and lumbar disc herniations. *Journal of Manipulative and Physiological Therapeutics* 19(19).

Eriksen, K. 1998. Management of cervical disc herniation with upper cervical chiropractic care. *Journal of Manipulative and Physiological Therapeutics* 21(1).

Esch, S. 1998. Case #2: Adjustive treatment for chronic respiratory ailment in a five-year-old. Case reports in chiropractic pediatrics. *American Chiropractic Association Journal of Chiropractic* (Dec.).

Fallon, J. 1991. The effects of chiropractic treatment on pregnancy and labor: a comprehensive study. *Proceedings of the World Chiropractic Congress,* 1991 :24–31.

Fallon, J.M. 1997. The role of the chiropractic adjustment in the care and treatment of 332 children with otitis media. *Journal of Clinical Chiropractic Pediatrics* 2(2):167–83.

Farley, Dixie. 1997. Bone builders: support your bones with healthy habits. *FDA Consumer Magazine* Sept.–Oct. http://www.webmd.com.

Faulkner, T.L., and L.E. Ward. 1994. Duchenne's muscular dystrophy: a chiropractic approach. *Chiropractic: The Journal of Chiropractic Research and Clinical Investigation* 9(3):76–80.

Feuling, Timothy J. 1999. *Chiropractic Works! Adjusting to a Higher Quality of Life.* [No location given]: Wellness Solutions.

Fidelibus, J. 1989. An overview of neuroimmunomodulation and a possible correlation with musculoskeletal system function. *Journal of Manipulative and Physiological Therapeutics* (Aug.).

Fortinopoulos, V. 1999. Scoliosis and subluxation. *International Chiropractic Pediatric Association* (Jul./Aug.).

Freitag, P. 1987. Expert testimony of Dr. Pertag, M.D., Ph.D., comparing results of two neighboring hospitals, stating that less painkillers needed during delivery if patient under chiropractic care. Testimony offered during trial in U.S. District Court Northern Illinois Eastern Division, No. 76C 3777.

Frequency of medical negligence in the hospital. 1991. *Journal Watch.* Feb. 8.

Frymann, V.M., R.D. Carney, and P. Springall. 1992. Effect of osteopathic medical management on neurologic development in children. *Journal of the American Osteopathic Association* 92:729–44.

Fulford, R.C., D.O. 1996. *Dr. Fulford's Touch of Life: The Healing Power of the Natural Life Force.* New York: Pocket Books.

Fysh, D.C. 1996. Chronic recurrent otitis media. *Journal of Clinical Chiropractic Pediatrics* 1(2):66–78.

Giesen, J.M., D.B. Center, and R.A. Leach. 1989. An evaluation of chiropractic manipulation as a treatment of hyperactivity in children. *Journal of Manipulative and Physiological Therapeutics* 12:353–63.

Giles, L.G., and R. Muller. 1999. Chronic spinal pain syndrome: a clinical pilot trial comparing acupuncture, a nonsteroidal anti-inflammatory drug (NSAID), and spinal manipulation. *Journal of Manipulative and Physiological Therapeutics* 22(6):376–81.

Gillespie, L., R. Bray, N. Levin, and R. Delamarter. 1991. Lumbar nerve root compression and interstitial cystitis—response to decompressive surgery. *British Journal of Neurology* 68:361–64.

Golden, L., and C. Van Egmond. 1994. Longitudinal clinical case study: multidisciplinary care of child with multiple functional and developmental disorders. *Journal of Manipulative and Physiological Therapeutics* 17(4):79.

Goldman, S.R. 1995. Subluxation location and correction (31-year-old with Crohn's disease). *Today's Chiropractic* (Jul./Aug.):70–74.

Goodman, R. 1992. Hypertension and the atlas subluxation complex. *Chiropractic: Journal of Chiropractic Research and Clinical Investigation* 8(2).

Graham, R.L., and R.A. Pistolese. 1997. An impairment rating analysis of asthmatic children under chiropractic care. *Journal of Vertebral Subluxation Research* 1(4).

Gutmann, G. 1990. Blocked atlantal nerve syndrome in infants and small children. *International Review of Chiropractic* 46(4):37. English translation of German paper published 1987 in *Manuelle Medizin.*

Hayward, R.A., M.D., and T.P. Hofer, M.D. 2001. Estimating hospital deaths due to medical errors: preventability is in the eye of the reviewer. *Journal of the American Medical Association* 286:415–20.

Healey, Mark A., M.D., Steven R. Shackford, M.D., Turner M. Osler, M.D., Frederick B. Rogers, M.D., and Elizabeth Burns, R.N., M.S., A.N.P. 2002. Complications in Surgical Patients (abstract). *Archives of Surgery* 137:611–618. http://www.jama.org.

Healthwise. 2002. Glucosamine and chondroitin: other treatments for osteoarthritis. *Health Guides A–Z,* http://www.webmd.com.

————. 2002. Osteoarthritis. *Health Guides A–Z,* http://www.webmd.com.

Hendelman, Walter J., M.D. 2000. *Atlas of Functional Neuroanatomy.* Boca Raton: CRC Press.

Hewitt, E.G. 1993. Chiropractic treatment of a 7-month-old with chronic constipation: a case report. *Chiropractic Technique* 5(3):101–3.

Homola, S., D.C. 1999. *Inside Chiropractic: A Patient's Guide.* Amherst, NY: Prometheus Books.

Hospers, L.A. 1992. EG and CEEG studies before and after upper cervical or SOT category 11 adjustment in children after heat trauma, in epilepsy, and in "hyperactivity." *Procedures of the National Conference on Chiropractic and Pediatrics (ICA)*:84–139.

Hurst, L.C., D. Weissberg, and R.E. Carroll. 1985. The relationship of the double crush syndrome (an analysis of 1,000 cases of carpal tunnel syndrome). *Journal of Hand Surgery* 10B:202.

Hurwitz, E.L., D.C., et al. 1998. The number of DC's and the percent of the population using chiropractic. *American Journal of Public Health* 88(5):771–76.

Iyengar, B.K.S. 1966. *Light on Yoga.* New York: Schocken Books.

Jaret, Peter. 2001. Turning the pyramid upside down. *WebMD Medical News,* Feb. 26. http://www.webmd.com.

Jarmel, M.E., J.L. Zatkin, E. Charuvastra, and W.E. Shell. 1995. Improvements of cardiac autonomic regulation following spinal manipulative therapy. Unpublished paper presented at the July Chiropractic Centennial event, Washington, D.C.

Kapandji, I.A. 1974. *The Physiology of the Joints, Volume Three: The Trunk and Vertebral Column* (second edition). New York: Churchill Livingston.

Kessinger, R. 1997. Changes in pulmonary function associated with upper cervical specific chiropractic care. *Journal of Vertebral Subluxation Research* 1(3):43–49.

Kirby, S.L. 1994. A case study: the effects of chiropractic on multiple sclerosis. *Chiropractic Research Journal* 3(1).

Klougart, N., N. Nilsson, and J. Jacobsen. 1989. Infantile colic treated by chiropractors: a prospective study of 316 cases. *Journal of Manipulative and Physiological Therapeutics* 12:281–88.

Kohn, Linda T., Janet M. Corrigan, and Molla S. Donaldson, eds. 2000. *To Err Is Human: Building a Safer Health System.* Washington, D.C.: Institute of Medicine.

Kokjohn, J., D.M. Schmid, J.J. Triano, and P.C. Brennan. 1992. The effect of spinal manipulation on pain and prostaglandin levels in women with primary dysmenorrhea. *Journal of Manipulative and Physiological Therapeutics* 15(5):279–85.

Koren, T., ed. 2000. *Chiropractic and Spinal Research,* 2000 Edition. Philadelphia: Koren Publications, Inc.

Korr, I.M. 1978. *The Neurobiologic Mechanisms in Manipulative Therapy.* New York: Plenum.

Kunau, P.L. 1998. Application of the Webster in-utero constraint technique: a case series. *Journal of Clinical Chiropractic Pediatrics* 3(1).

LaBarbera, J.A. 1998. Tourette syndrome, case study. *International Chiropractic Pediatric Association Newsletter,* Utica, NY, Mar./Apr.

Lang, J., D.C. 1987. The way of stillness. In *The Heart of the Healer,* ed. D. Church and Dr. A. Sherr. New York: Aslan Publishing.

Larsen, William J. 1998. *Essentials of Human Embryology,* New York: Churchill Livingston.

Lauro, A., and B. Mouch. Chiropractic effects on athletic ability. *Chiropractic: The Journal of Chiropractic Research and Clinical Investigation* 6:84–87.

LeBoeuf, C., P. Brown, A. Herman, K. Leembruggen, D. Walton, and T.C. Crisp. 1991. Chiropractic care of children with nocturnal enuresis: a prospective outcome study. *Journal of Manipulative and Physiological Therapeutics* 14(2):110–15.

Lee, G., and C.D. Jenson. 1998. Remission of hepatocellular carcinoma in a patient under chiropractic care: a case report. *Journal of Vertebral Subluxation Research* 2(3):n.p.

Levine, Jeff. 2000. Experts seek to understand epidemic of medical errors: summit aims to set research agenda for reducing death, injury toll. *WebMD Medical News,* Sept. 11. http://www.webmd.com.

Lewit, K. 1991. *Manipulative Therapy and Rehabilitation of the Locomotor System.* Oxford: Butterworth-Heineman.

Liebl, N., and L. Butler. 1990. A chiropractic approach to the treatment of dysmenorrhea. *Journal of Manipulative and Physiological Therapeutics* (Feb.):101–6.

Lipton, B.H. 1998. The Evolving Science of Chiropractic Philosophy. *Today's Chiropractic* 27(5):16–19.

———. 1999. The Evolving Science of Chiropractic Philosophy. Part II. *Today's Chiropractic* 28(6):21–30.

Loomis, H., D.C. 1995. Introducing a "vital" subject. *The Chiropractic Journal* (Sept.). Online edition, http://www.worldchiropracticalliance.org.

———. 1995. No "magic bullets." *The Chiropractic Journal* (Nov.). Online edition, http://www.worldchiropracticalliance.org.

———. 1995. The concept of homeostasis. *The Chiropractic Journal* (Dec.). Online edition, http://www.worldchiropracticalliance.org.

———. 1996. The chiropractic model and digestive disorders. *The Chiropractic Journal* (Feb.). Online edition, http://www.worldchiropracticalliance.org.

————. 1996. Going beyond patchwork. *The Chiropractic Journal* (Mar.). Online edition, http://www.worldchiropracticalliance. org.

————. 1997. Nutrition, digestion and chiropractic. *The Chiropractic Journal* (Nov.). Online edition, http://www.worldchiropracticalliance.org.

————. 1999. Protein. *The Chiropractic Journal* (May). Online edition, http://www.worldchiropracticalliance.org.

————. 2001. The large intestine and lumbar spine. *The Chiropractic Journal* (Jan.). Online edition, http://www.worldchiropracticalliance.org.

————. 2001. Homeostasis: The deviations. *The Chiropractic Journal* (Mar.). Online edition, http://www.worldchiropracticalliance.org.

————. 2001. Subluxation: cause or effect? *The Chiropractic Journal* (Sept.). Online edition, http://www.worldchiropracticalliance.org.

————. 2001. One disease? *The Chiropractic Journal* (Nov.). Online edition, http://www.worldchiropracticalliance.org.

Lown, Bernard, M.D. 1996. *The Lost Art of Healing.* New York: Houghton Mifflin Company.

Marko, R.B. 1994. Bed-wetting: two case studies. *Chiropractic Pediatrics* 1(1).

Marko, S. 1994. Case study: the effect of chiropractic care on an infant with problems of constipation. *Chiropractic Pediatrics* 1(3).

Martin, Sean. 2000. Dueling diets: creators of popular diets find little common ground on healthy eating. *WebMD Medical News,* Feb. 24. http://www.webmd.com.

Mathews, J.A., et al. 1987. Back pain and sciatica: controlled trials of manipulation, traction, sclerosant and epidural injections. *British Journal of Rheumatology* 26:416–23.

Mathews, M.O., and E. Thomas. 1993. A pilot study of applied kinesiology in helping children with learning disabilities. *British Osteopathic Journal* 12.

Mayer, J.W., et al. 1976. Brain stem compression in rheumatoid arthritis. *Journal of the American Medical Association* 236(18) (November 1).

McCoy, H.G., and M. McCoy. 1997. A multiple parameter assessment of whiplash injury patients undergoing subluxation-based chiropractic care: a retrospective study. *Journal of Vertebral Subluxation Research* 1(3).

McGill, L., D.C. 1997. *The Chiropractor's Health Book.* New York: Three Rivers Press.

McGuiness, J., B. Vicenzino, and A. Wright. 1997. Influence of a cervical mobilization technique on respiratory and cardiovascular function. *Manual Therapy* 2(4):216–20.

McKnight, M.E., and K.F. DeBoer. 1988. Preliminary study of blood pressure changes in normotensive subjects undergoing chiropractic care. *Journal of Manipulative and Physiological Therapeutics* 11:261–66.

Miller, W.D. 1975. Treatment of visceral disorders by manipulative therapy. In *The Research Status of Spinal Manipulative Therapy,* M. Goldstein, ed. Bethesda, MD: Department of Health, Education, and Welfare.

Murphy, D.R. 1994. Diagnosis and manipulative treatment in diabetic polyneuropathy and its relation to intertarsal joint dysfunction. *Journal of Manipulative and Physiological Therapeutics* 17:29–37.

Murray, Michael T., N.D. 2002. *The Pill Book Guide to Natural Medicines.* New York: Bantam Books.

Nall, S.K. 1982. The role of specific manipulation towards alleviating abnormalities in body mechanics and restoration of spinal motion. *Journal of Manipulative and Physiological Therapeutics* 5:11–15.

National Heart, Lung, and Blood Institute. 1998. *Facts about the DASH Diet.* NIH Publication No. 98-4082. http://www.nhlbi.nih.gov/health/public/heart/hbp/dash/dashbody.htm. On http://www.webmd.com.

————. 1999. *Cardiovascular Information for Patients and the General Public. How to Prevent High Blood Pressure.* http://www.nhlbi.nih.gov/health/public/heart/hbp/prevhpb/index.htm. On http://www.webmd.com.

National Institute of Allergy and Infectious Diseases. 1990. Fact sheet: food allergy and intolerances. Rev. Jan. 1999. *Health Topics A–Z,* http://www.webmd.com.

National Institutes of Health. 1994. *Alternative Medicine: Expanding Medical Horizons. A Report to the National Institutes of Health and Alternative Medical Systems and Practices in the United States.* NIH Publication No. 94-066. On http://www.webmd.com.

Nelson, C.F., G. Bronfort, R. Evans, et al. 1998. The efficacy of spinal manipulation, amitriptyline and the combination of both therapies for prophylaxis of migraine headache. *Journal of Manipulative and Physiological Therapeutics* 21(8):511–19.

Nelson, W.A. 1989. Diabetes mellitus: two case reports. *Chiropractic Technique* 1:37–40.

Newberg, A., M.D., E. D'Aquili, M.D., and Vince Rause. 2001. *Why God Won't Go Away: Brain Science and the Biology of Belief.* New York: Ballantine Books.

Nilsson, D.C., et al. 1997. Study of the effect of spinal manipulation on cervicogenic headaches. *Journal of Manipulative and Physiological Therapeutics* 20(5):326–30.

Noll, D.R., J. Shores, P.N. Bryman, and E.V. Masterson. 1999. Adjustive osteopathic manipulative treatment in the elderly hospitalized with pneumonia: a pilot study. *Journal of the American Osteopathic Association* 99(3):143–46.

Null, G. 1999. *Gary Null's Ultimate Anti-Aging Program.* New York: Broadway Books.

Nyiendo, J., and E. Olsen. 1988. Characteristics of 217 children attending a chiropractic college teaching clinic. *Journal of Manipulative and Physiological Therapeutics* 11(2):780–84.

Ochs, Ridgely. 2001. Posture added to RSI equation. *Los Angeles Times,* Health section, August 27.

Osterbauer, P.J., and A.W. Fuhr. 1992. Treatment of chronic sciatica by mechanical force, manually assisted, short lever adjusting, and a video assisted stretching program: a quantitative case report. *Proceedings of the Consortium for Chiropractic Research and Education.* Palm Springs, CA.

Otte, A., T.M. Ettlin, E.U. Nitzsche, K. Wachter, S. Hoegerle, G.H. Simon, L. Fierz, E. Moser, and J. Mueller-Brand. 1997. PET and SPECT in whiplash syndrome: a new approach to a forgotten brain? *Journal of Neurology, Neurosurgery, and Psychiatry* 63:368 72.

Palkhivala, Alison. 2001. Is your job a pain in the back? *WebMD Medical News*, Jul. 2. http://www.webmd.com.

———. 2001. Shaping a better food pyramid guide. *Food and Nutrition*, Sept. 17. http://www.webmd.com.

Palmer, B.J. 1934. *The Subluxation Specific—The Adjustment Specific: An Exposition of the Cause of All Disease*. Spartanburg, SC: Sherman College of Straight Chiropractic.

———. 1950. *Up from Below the Bottom*. Spartanburg, SC: Sherman College of Straight Chiropractic.

Palmer, D.D. 1910. *The Chiropractor's Adjuster*. Portland, OR: Portland Printing House.

Peterson, K.B. 1997. The effects of spinal manipulation on the intensity of emotional arousal in phobic subjects exposed to a threat stimulus: a randomized, controlled, double-blind clinical trial. *Journal of Manipulative and Physiological Therapeutics* 20(9):602–6.

Phillips, David P., and Charlene C. Bredder. 2002. Morbidity and mortality from medical errors: an increasingly serious public health problem (abstract). *Annual Review of Public Health* 23:135–50. http://www.jama.org.

Pikalov, A.A., and V.V. Kharin. 1994. Use of spinal manipulative therapy in the treatment of duodenal ulcer: a pilot study. *Journal of Manipulative and Physiological Therapeutics* 17(5):310.

Pistolese, R.A. 1998. Risk assessment of neurological and/or vertebrobasilar complications in the pediatric chiropractic patient. (Risk of complications in pediatric patients under chiropractic care.) *Journal of Vertebral Subluxation Research* 2(2):73–81.

Porter, R. 1997. *The Greatest Benefit to Mankind: A Medical History of Humanity*. New York: W. W. Norton & Company.

Potthoff, S., B. Penwell, and J. Wolf. 1993. Panic attacks and the chiropractic adjustment: a case report. *American Chiropractic Association Journal of Chiropractic* 30 (Dec.):26–28.

Purse, F.M. 1966. Manipulative therapy of upper respiratory tract infections in children. *Journal of the American Osteopathic Association* 65(9):964–72.

Rause, V. 2001. The biology of belief. *Los Angeles Times Magazine*, Jul. 15.

Roberts, J.M. 1993. *History of the World*, New York: Oxford University Press.

Rondberg, T.A., D.C. 1996. *Chiropractic First: The Fastest Growing Healthcare Choice . . . Before Drugs or Surgery*. Chandler, AZ: The Chiropractic Journal.

Rondberg, T.A., D.C., and T.J. Feuling. 1998. Chiropractic: Compassion and Expectation. Chandler, AZ: The Chiropractic Journal.

Rothschild, Jeffrey M., M.D., M.P.H., David W. Bates, M.D., M.Sc., and Lucian L. Leape, M.D. 2000. Preventable medical injuries in older patients (abstract). *Archives of Internal Medicine* 160:2717–28. http://www.jama.org.

Sandeful, R., and E. Adams. 1987. The effect of chiropractic adjustments on the behavior of autistic children: a case review. *American Chiropractic Association Journal of Chiropractic* 21 (Dec.):5.

Scarborough, J. 2001. Hippocrates. *World Book Online American Edition.* Chicago, IL: World Book, Inc.

Schmidt, I.C. 1982. Osteopathic manipulative therapy as a primary factor in the management of upper, middle and pararespiratory infections. *Journal of the American Osteopathic Association* (Feb.):2388.

Schneier, M., and R. Burns. 1989. Atlanto-occipital hypermobility in sudden infant death syndrome. Report released by Association for Research in Chiropractic. Apr.

Schwarzbein, D., M.D., and Nancy Deville. 1999. *The Schwarzbein Principle: The Truth About Losing Weight, Being Healthy and Feeling Younger.* Deerfield Beach, FL: Health Communications, Inc.

Sears, B., with B. Lawren. 1995. *The Zone: A Dietary Road Map to Lose Weight Permanently.* New York: HarperCollins.

Selano, J.L., B.C. Hightower, B. Pfleger, et al. 1994. The effects of specific upper cervical adjustment on the CD4 counts of HIV positive patients. *Chiropractic Research Journal* 3(1):32–39.

Shara, K. 1999. Bell's palsy, a chiropractic case study. *Sacrooccipital Resource Society International* 11(2):n.p.

Shatz, Mary Pullig, M.D. 1992. *Back Care Basics.* Berkeley: Rodmell Press.

Shekelle, P., M.D., Ph.D. 1997. After lower back pain, neck pain and headaches the most common reasons for providing spinal manipulation. *Journal of Spinal Disorders* 10(3):223–28.

Silverman, Harold M., Pharm.D., Joseph Romano, and Gary Elmer. 1985. *The Vitamin Book.* New York: Bantam Books.

Sportelli, L., D.C. 2000. *A Natural Method of Health Care: Introduction to Chiropractic.* Palmerton, PA: Practice Makers Products, Inc.

State Supervisor of Chiropractors of Kentucky. 1931. Chiropractic success in a reform school. Report in connection with Kentucky Houses of Reform, Greendale, Kentucky. Lexington, KY, Dec. 1.

Stein, Loren, and Rob Waters. 2000. RX errors on the rise. *WebMD Medical News,* Oct. 23. Updated Apr. 5, 2002. http://www.webmd.com.

Stephens, D., and M. Gorman. 1996. Does "normal" vision improve with spinal manipulation? *Journal of Manipulative and Physiological Therapeutics* 19:415–18.

Stephenson, R.W. 1948. *Chiropractic Textbook.* Davenport, IA: The Palmer School of Chiropractic.

Stress management. 2001. *Health Guide A–Z.* Updated May 11. http://www.webmd.com.

Stude, D.E., and T. Mick. 1993. Clinical presentation of a patient with multiple sclerosis and response to manual chiropractic adjustive therapies. *Journal of Manipulative and Physiological Therapeutics* 16:595–600.

Talbot, M. 1991. *The Holographic Universe.* New York: HarperPerennial.

Terrett, A.G., and R.F. Gorman. 1995. The eye, the cervical spine, and spinal manipulative therapy: a review of the literature. *Chiropractic Technique* 7(2).

Thomas, Lewis. 1974. *Lives of a Cell: Notes of a Biology Watcher.* New York: Penguin Books.

————. 1979. *The Medusa and the Snail: More Notes of a Biology Watcher.* New York: Viking Press.

————. 1983. *The Youngest Science: Notes of a Medicine Watcher.* New York: Viking Press.

————. 1992. *The Fragile Species.* New York: Charles Scribner's Sons.

Thomason, P.R., B.L. Fisher, et al. 1979. Effectiveness of spinal manipulative therapy in treatment of primary dysmenorrhea: a pilot study. *Journal of Manipulative and Physiological Therapeutics* 2:140–45.

Tools for changing your diet. 2001. *Health Topics A–Z,* Apr. 16. http://www.webmd.com.

Troyanovich, S.J., D.D. Harrison, and D.E. Harrison. 1999. Low back pain and the lumbar intervertebral disk: clinical consideration for the doctor of chiropractic. *Journal of Manipulative and Physiological Therapeutics* 22(2):96–104.

Unger, J., S. Sweat, S. Flanagan, and S. Chudowski. 1993. An effect of sacrooccipital technique on blood pressure. In *Proceedings of the International Conference on Spinal Manipulation.*

Van Breda, W.M., and J.M. Van Breda. 1989. A comparative study of the health status of children raised under the health care models of chiropractic and allopathic medicine. *Journal of Chiropractic Research* (Summer):101–3.

Wagner, T., J. Owen, E. Malone, and K. Mann. 1996. Irritable bowel syndrome and spinal manipulation: a case report. *Chiropractic Technique* 7:139–40.

Walsh, M., and B. Polus. 1999. The frequency of positive common spinal clinical examination findings in a sample of premenstrual syndrome sufferers. *Journal of Manipulative and Physiological Therapeutics* 22(4):n.p.

Walton, E.V. 1975. The effects of chiropractic treatment on students with learning and behavioral impairments due to neurological dysfunction. *International Review of Chiropractic* 29:4–5, 24–26.

Ward, L. 1995. The role of chiropractic in the management of degenerative disease cases. *Today's Chiropractic* (Jul./Aug.).

Warner, S.P., and T.M. Warner. 1999. Case report: autism and chronic otitis media. *Today's Chiropractic* (May/June).

Webster, L. 1994. Hip dysplasia in seven-day-old infant: case study. *Chiropractic Showcase Magazine* 2(5).

————. 1994. Stuttering, hyperactivity, slow learner, retarded growth: case study. *Chiropractic Showcase Magazine* 2 (5).

————. 1995. Inability to conceive: two case histories. *International Chiropractic Pediatric Association Newsletter* (Nov.).

Weil, A., M.D. 1995. *Spontaneous Healing: How to Discover and Enhance Your Body's Natural Ability to Maintain and Heal Itself.* New York: Alfred A. Knopf.

Wendel, P. 1998. ADHD—a multiple case study. *International Chiropractic Pediatric Association* (Mar./Apr.).

Whittingham, W., W.B. Ellis, and T.P. Molyneux. 1994. The effect of manipulation (toggle recoil technique) for headaches with upper cervical joint dysfunction: a pilot study. *Journal of Manipulative and Physiological Therapeutics* 17(6):369–75.

Wiberg, J.M.M., J. Norsteen, and N. Nilsson. 1999. The short-term effect of spinal manipulation in the treatment of infantile colic: a randomized controlled clinical trial with a blinded observer. *Journal of Manipulative and Physiological Therapeutics* 22(8):517–22.

Winsor, H. 1921. The prevalence of minor curvatures and deformities of the spine in man, also in other vertebrates. *The Medical Times* 49 (Oct.):237–39.

————. 1921. The evidence of the association, in dissected cadavers, of visceral disease with vertebrae deformities of the same sympathetic segments: Sympathetic segmental disturbances—II. *The Medical Times* 49 (Nov.):267–71.

Wittler, N.A. 1992. Chiropractic approach to premenstrual syndrome. *Chiropractic: The Journal of Chiropractic Research and Clinical Investigation* 8:22–29.

Woo, C.C. 1993. Post-traumatic myelopathy following high jump: a pilot case of spinal manipulation. *Journal of Manipulative and Physiological Therapeutics* 16(5):336–41.

Wood, John N., ed. 2000. *Molecular Basis of Pain Induction.* New York: Wiley-Liss.

Wrightson, P., V. McGinn, and D. Gronwell. 1995. Mild head injury in preschool children: evidence that it can be associated with a persisting cognitive defect. *Journal of Neurology, Neurosurgery, and Psychiatry* 59:375–80.

Yates, R.G., D.L. Lamping, N.L. Abram, and C. Wright. 1988. Effects of chiropractic treatment on blood pressure and anxiety. *Journal of Manipulative and Physiological Therapeutics* 11:484–88.

Zukav, G. 1979. *The Dancing Wu Li Masters.* New York: William Morrow.

ACKNOWLEDGMENTS

While this book is the result of years of experience in my chosen profession of chiropractic, it could not have come into being without the help and support of many people, both personally and professionally. First and foremost I wish to thank my wife, Susan, a remarkable woman, not only for her proofreading and her insightful contributions to the dietary aspects of this book, but also for her enduring support on every possible level of my wild optimism and endless dreams. Thanks to my daughter, Jennifer, for allowing me to be her friend as well as her parent, and for her love and support of me in both those roles. To my mom and dad, Marye and Larry Lenarz, for their kindness and generosity—and allowing me to stay with them in the desert while I worked on writing this book. Thanks also to Mom and Dad Klemmer for their friendship and support throughout the years.

I could not have taken the time to write this book if I didn't have the backing of the people who work with me at the Health First clinic. To all the staff, and especially to Sheila, the strength at the front office, Brooke at our Kirkland office, and Molly, our public relations genius, thank you. Special acknowledgment must go to the chiropractors who have worked with me over the years. Dr. Chris Wolff and Dr. Darren White, as well as Drs. Chris DeGeorge, Cliff Fisher, and Todd Hubbard—I consider you close friends and I thank you for allowing me the time to travel, speak, write, and teach.

In my continuing study of the field of chiropractic, I have had the good fortune to associate with some of the best and brightest in our profession. Some of the "heroes" who have contributed to my growth and understanding of chiropractic include Drs. Thom and Betty Gelardi, founders of Sherman College of Straight Chiropractic, and Dr. Guy Riekeman, President of Palmer Colleges. Thanks also to Dr. Weldon Muncy and Mrs. Millie Muncy, who took the time to train me and countless others in the path of Blair Upper Cervical chiropractic, and to Dr. William Blair and his remarkable wife, Dottie. My teachers at Sherman College of Straight Chiropractic left an enduring mark on my professional and personal life, especially Drs. Perry Rush, Anthony Duke, Sheldon Clayton, David Koch, Leroy Moore, and Gary Vidrine. I am fortunate to count Drs. Noel Lloyd and Lee Newman as my teachers as well as my friends and business associates.

A special word must be said about the contributions to chiropractic made by Dr. Tedd Koren and Dr. Terry Rondberg. Dr. Koren's fervor for and dedication to chiropractic is renowned throughout our profession, and his compilations of research sources were invaluable in the preparation of this book. Dr. Rondberg is the founder of the World Chiropractic Alliance and author of numerous books and articles on the history, philosophy, and practice of chiropractic. He is a tireless advocate for chiropractic care and a powerful voice for our profession. I also wish to acknowledge Malik Slosberg for his ongoing compilation of scientific research that validates the chiropractic premise and clinical experience. In addition, I am most grateful to have permission from Bruce Lipton, Ph.D., to draw on his powerful and innovative work on the science of chiropractic philosophy.

In my years as a practitioner of chiropractic, I have been fortunate to encounter several conventional medical doctors with whom I have had some stimulating dialogues about modern medicine. In their intellectual openness and their willingness to think of the good of the patient above all else, Drs. Ed Hanzelick, John Horton, Anil Daya, and Henry Warszawski (M.D.'s all) have shown me the true heart of medicine and how it is really meant to be practiced. And although I have not met them personally, I wish to acknowledge the contributions made by Drs. Deepak Chopra, Andrew Weil, and Bernie Siegel for the foundations they have laid for a more sane and safe health care model.

Getting a book published requires focus and stamina, and if you're lucky, you have a team of people who help you get the job done right. I cannot say enough about Carol Roth, my friend and agent, who walked me through revision after revision of my original book outline and proposal. Thanks also to the people at the Maui Writers Conference who brought us together. My co-writer, Victoria St. George of Just Write, has been a remarkable and hardworking partner. I am also grateful for the vision and deft editing of Toni Burbank, my editor at Bantam Books. In fact, the whole team at Bantam has been brilliant and enjoyable to work with. Thanks to you all—and I hope you enjoy the results of our collaboration as much as I do.

Finally, I would like to thank all the hundreds of thousands of patients who choose to make chiropractic a part of their ongoing health care, especially those whom I myself have treated in my fifteen-plus years as a chiropractor. Their stories of the journey from pain to relief, injury to healing, disease to radiant health have enriched my life beyond measure. I honor and value my patients' trust, and I will continue to do everything I can to ensure that more people everywhere reap the benefits of chiropractic care.

ABOUT THE AUTHOR

Michael Lenarz received his Doctor of Chiropractic Degree from Sherman College of Straight Chiropractic in Spartanburg, South Carolina, where he received the B. J. Palmer Philosophical Distinction Award. He is an extension faculty member for Sherman College and for Logan Chiropractic College in Kansas City, Missouri, and a committee member for the Blair Chiropractic Society. Dr. Lenarz has been in practice for 15 years and operates three chiropractic offices in Seattle and northern Washington. Dr. Lenarz is also a practice management consultant for chiropractors and speaks at chiropractic events nationwide.

Victoria St. George is a writer and editor living in Santa Monica, California. She is also partner in Just Write, a literary services firm with offices in California and Virginia.